Dear Sandi, 3/12

Embrace your

(Rachel)

A LEAF FALLS....A BUD BLOSSOMS

ONE CODEPENDENT'S JOURNEY

TO HEAL THE WOUNDED SOUL

RACHEL LIEBERMAN

A Leaf Falls...A Bud Blossoms

by Rachel Lieberman

Published by: My Inner Child Creations
Rachel Lieberman Suite 144
3840 W. Hillsboro Blvd.
Deerfield Beach, Fl 33442

Edited by: Arleen Baron

Cover photography by: Custom Photo Images

Printed by: Universal Graphics and Printing
North Palm Beach, Fl

ISBN: 0-9657142-0-9 $13.95

"Example is not the main thing in influencing others. It is the only thing."

Albert Schweitzer

DEDICATION

TO DON MOORE, L.C.S.W., WHOSE EXAMPLE

LIGHTS MY WAY ON THE PATH TO RECOVERY

BUTTERFLIES

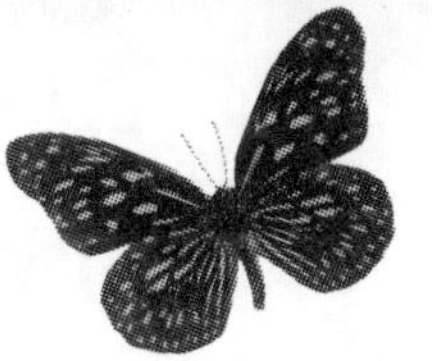

Butterflies are free! To me, they represent many things. They reflect G-d's awesome beauty. The symmetrical balance in their wing designs send me the message of living a more balanced life. I feel the freedom to be me with spirit in flight. Butterflies do a ballet, as they flit and flow through the air.

The evolution of the butterfly from a caterpillar is one of the most miraculous stories of metamorphosis that I have known! Caterpillars serve their place in nature's evolutionary process. They do their job and continue forward. The cocoon becomes its haven of privacy and development. During this stage, the miracle begins. Slowly and delicately, G-d becomes the sculptor of this fragile and magnificent creation. The struggle to emerge from the cocoon is vital and without it, the butterfly will soon die after its emergence.

The butterfly represents change and metamorphosis in my life physically, emotionally and spiritually. I feel that I have been given a second change to be beautiful and real!

It was hard work breaking out of the chrysalis. I stayed wrapped in G-d's cocoon of love and emerged into the sunlight of recovery. The butterfly has been my ongoing sign and symbol of that change in my life today. Now, in having patience to wait for my wings to dry, I can begin to soar!

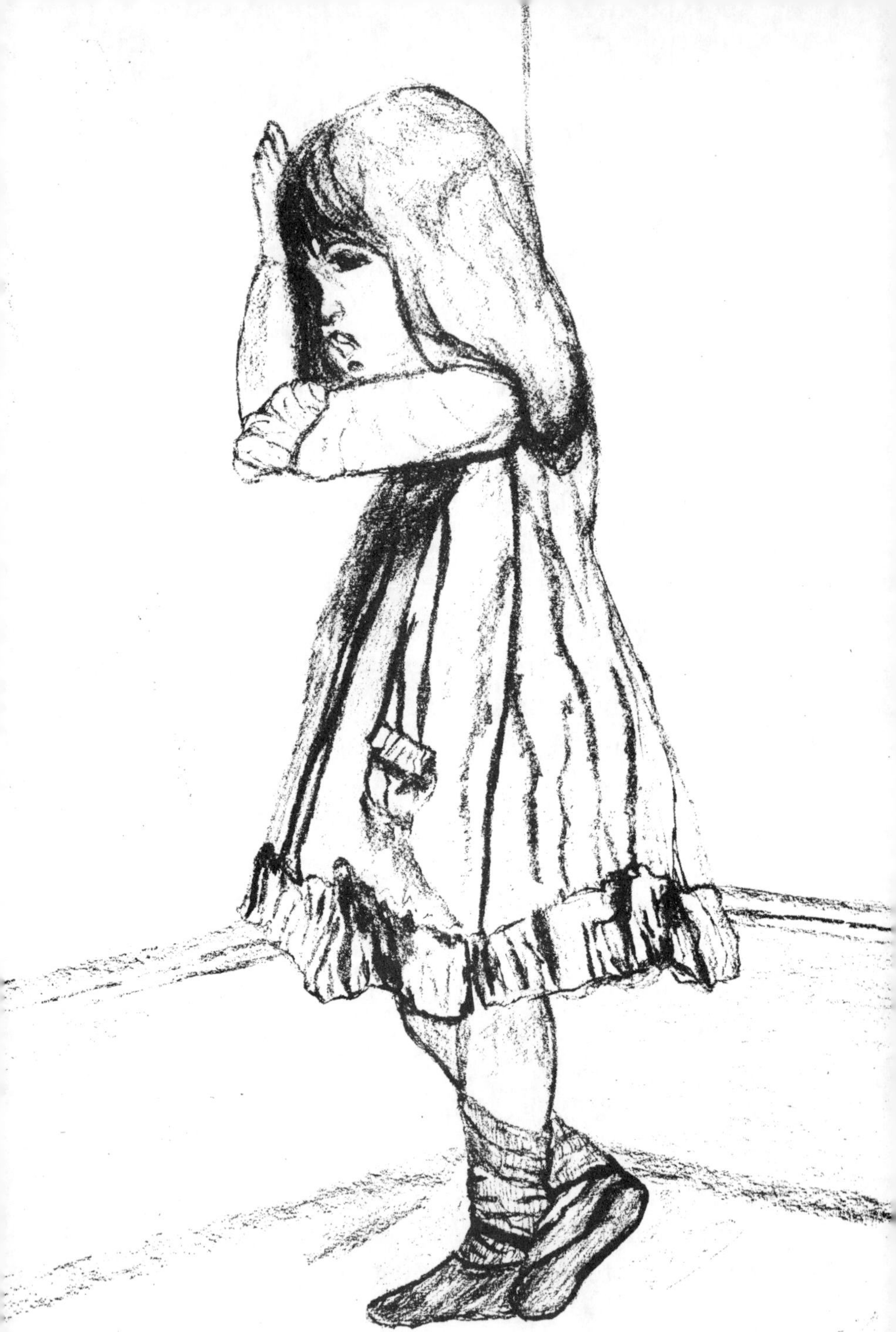

Please help me, help me.......
Drawing created by Debra Jermyn, Woodway, Texas

FOREWORD

Rachel invited me to write this forward because she knows I love her and because I was there when the seed for this book started to sprout. Sometime after we started to write a newsletter together, I noticed that words flew out of Rachel's typewriter and onto the page in the form of poetry. Rachel was constantly sharing a new poem.

Once a month Rachel and I would sit in my computer room to put our newsletter together. There she confided to me her strong desire to publish her poems in a book of her own making. Though Rachel felt that she might really do this someday, she asked, "Do you really think I can write a book?" "You read astrology charts, look at mine and see what it says."

I believe that a person's individual gifts and potentials as well as some of their life's conflicts can be seen in their natal or birth chart. Rachel's chart showed a strong talent for writing and an even stronger need for self-communication. It also showed her individual gifts and potentials that would be hers, if she met the challenges of her life. Each of us come into the world with gifts to be shared with others. This is what I found in Rachel's chart.

My special friend Rachel is always searching out the meaning of life. She finds that meaning from time to time and when she does she is able to convey her thoughts and feelings to others. Her spirit is an inspiration to many who come into contact with her. She finds herself and meaning in life by working through great emotional strife.

A tremendous desire to fight depression brought Rachel into the Twelve Step community. This book is about the spiritual tools she learned to use; to guide the choices she needed to make to change her life. It's about the help she got from therapy and her friends as she reached out to them with honesty. It's about the development of her faith and trust in others as well as in herself. It's about her letting go of childhood needs and desires. It's the story of how Rachel changed and how she has come to experience pleasure and a deep contentment in her life.

It is my hope that Rachel's written words will be an inspiration to her readers as her life is to her friends. You, the reader, are invited to enjoy these pages. You are free to take as your own whatever moves you and leave the rest.

Judith Goldstein
Aventura, Florida, 1996

INTRODUCTION

For me, writing this book feels like someone weaving a beautiful and very intricate tapestry of fine fabric. The design must be very carefully planned and it must be pleasing to the senses and appeal to the person choosing it to adorn their home or office. In the case of a book, it must also be an integral part of the author's total energy experience.

This is my first endeavor, on my recovering journey to wholeness, to share publicly in writing, the amazing process and experience of finding my Higher Power, my inner child, my heart and my soul. The experience of recovering and healing from the devastating disease of codependency and discovering all the doors that have opened for me to inner peace, is my message to you, the reader, in this my first publication.

Many codependent experts around the country agree that this very toxic disease is a true loss of self; the loss of feeling anything positive about one's self-esteem or self-worth. It is basically the loss of dealing well with relationships and feelings in our lives. Three of the culprits that cause this to happen are usually shame, guilt and fear. These three stem from all the severe dysfunctions of our families of origin; the seeds of the disease being there from birth and playing themselves out.

In the past six years, I have noticed that self-help sections of the better known bookstores around the country have grown enormously. For me and many others, it was the "Oprahs" of the television world that began to open our hearts and minds to a better understanding of what makes us tick. Slowly, the skeleton closets began to open and people had the courage to sit before millions and talk about their most inner pain and dysfunction! The John Bradshaws and the Bernie Siegels of the world offer us a wealth of possibilities for emotional balance and well-being, when we are ready. In talking about family dysfunction, recovery speakers also refer to the fog and trance that we many times experience before ever finding our way to the doors of recovery and discovery.

The Twelve Step Program originates from Alcoholics Anonymous back in the 1930's. It takes us step by step from acknowledging our issues to letting go of them where appropriate and making amends to all we have harmed by taking a moral inventory of ourselves.

This book, sharing my experience, strength and hope was inspired by my Higher Power and all the amazing support people in my life today. Having been given such a special gift of a healing journey, how could I not share it with you? In this book, **A Leaf Falls, A Bud Blossoms**, perhaps a clearer definition of the new household word, "codependency" will emerge for you, as you browse or are reading through these pages. Don't be surprised if the meaning of the title jumps right out for you, "as big as life"!

ACKNOWLEDGMENTS

Three years ago I felt a calling to write and share my experience, strength and hope with others. It was a year and a half later that I actually took pen to paper to begin this manuscript. It has been my greatest joy to create this first book, as a new author. There are so many to thank for their encouragement, support and help!

To G-d, my Higher Power, who guides and protects my soul with healing and spirituality.

My parents, who always did the very best job that they knew how to do for me.

My dear and loving husband for all his support each and every step of the way in all of life's events.

Dr. Reynold Stein, M.D., for his concern and help at the onset of my recovering process.

Melanie Kaleky and Rena Rantz, two soul friends, who invited me to my first therapy group. For adult children of dysfunctional families, at Don's office back in 1991.

Karen and Jay Okrent for giving me my first Bradshaw tape on shame. That tape was my first glimmer into understanding what might have happened to me in the past.

Rabbi/Dr. Jean-Claude Klein, Phy.D., for taking me to my very first Twelve-Step meeting and becoming my sponsor and friend.

Rabbi Simcha Freedman, over a ten year period, has been a beacon of spiritual support to me and my family, including experiencing my Bat-Mitzvah at the age of forty-three.

Recovery speaker, John Bradshaw, whose book, **Healing The Shame That Binds You**, truly opened my eyes early on in recovery to my dysfunctional family of origin.

Don Moore, L.C.S.W., to whom I dedicated this book, for his caring and hard work and constant encouragement that I can become that beautiful person that I was meant to be. For a long time, I stayed in denial, kicking and screaming all the way, until his therapeutic "magic" began to take hold.

Ken Spaziano, my CODA sponsor for three years is a spiritual inspiration to me on this journey.

Bob Singer, my message therapist, whose marvelous therapeutic talents have helped me heal and find my quiet within. I thank you.

"My family of choice", who give me ongoing support and love on this beautiful journey.

Glen Goodman, a therapist from Caron Foundation in Pennsylvania, who helped me to work through painful issues during my stay there.

Judy Sorge, my mamogram tech, for all the understanding and love she always extends to me. We will be "best friends forever".

Dr. Robert Derhagopian, M.D., whose professional and surgical expertise helped me to make my journey through lumpectomy and mastectomy, so much easier. I knew that G-d had lead me to just the right place.

Connie Goldstein, M.D., for offering me her medical assistance after my breast surgery.

Dr. Arnold Blaustein, M.D., my oncologist, for always giving me constant encouragement that there is "life after cancer".

Dr. Bernie Siegel, M.D., who was in South Florida two and a half years ago and helped me tremendously at his cancer seminar to process my needs and fears of having a breast implant.

Dr. Stephen Goldberg, M.D. and his wife, Harriet, for their help and suggestions to promote this book.

My friend, Paula Siegel and Dr. Jacob Elefant, D.D.S., who first helped me to begin accepting the anesthesia process before the lumpectomy.

Judy Goldstein, a very dear recovery friend who so generously offered to write the foreword with such joy!

Dr. Brian Greer, M.D., of the Center for Preventative Psychiatry. For his professional support and concern for my recovery.

Merrilee Middleton, Phy.D., of the Center for Group Counseling for all her efforts to impart the Rogerian way to all of us at the facilitator's workshop at the center and Wednesday morning supervisory meetings.

Lorraine Wilby, director of the Palm Beach Crisis Information Hotline, for all her help to become a crisis hotline volunteer.

Linda Kanter, of Hospice by the Sea, for all her encouragement and support, when I became a Hospice volunteer.

To all my personal friends in and out of recovery, I thank you all for your unconditional caring and love as I work each day on my journey to wholeness.

Dennis Beck of Universal Graphics and Printing, who took me under his wing as a new author and helped me to learn the ropes in preparing my book for print.

Kelly Phillips, Author of **Diary of an Anorexic**, for all her suggestions and help when I first began to write this book. Dr. Steven Goldberg, D.D.S., for his patience and understanding in helping me overcome my life long fears of dentistry.

Pete and Addie Lorber of Custom Photo Images, for all their help preparing the cover.

Elizabeth Caparros and Barbara Collins from The Counseling Centre in Boca Raton who have given me further enlightenment on my journey.

Arleen Baron, for her tremendous patience editing this book, it was an act of love.

Vin Cundari, my high school English and Journalism teacher, for all her caring and support through thick and thin. We have been soul friends for 40 years now.

Regina Moran for her untiring efforts and work to prepare my manuscript and redo it with me over and over again. Thank you.

Gertrude Edelman and John Sweeting, Principal and Vice Principal at school for all their ongoing support always.

To all those who contributed to Chapter Eight and your magnificent poetry, I thank you.

I truly appreciate the many people who gave me their continued encouragement to make this book a reality!

TABLE OF CONTENTS

"Every man has the right to risk his own life in order to save it."

Jean-Jacques Rousseau

DARKNESS BEFORE THE DAWN

CHAPTER I

Setting the stage
Finding Help
Opening up to heal

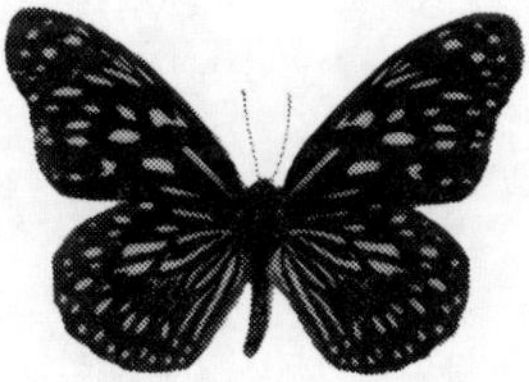

CHAPTER I

SETTING THE STAGE

I believe that I had a calling, not only to write and share this first volume with you, the reader, but, also to find my way into a life-long commitment to rebirth my soul with the recovering process. I knew something was very wrong for me when I was quite young, however, I wasn't able to define it back then as a small child. Childhood is a time of innocence; it is that time of absolute wondrous discovery of the world around us. At the time, I did not understand why it wasn't such a wondrous experience for me, as those younger, very difficult, years came along one by one.

It was Thanksgiving Day, 1939, the day I made my debut into this world. It was not the best of times; it was the worst of times. World War II had begun just a few months before. I was the sixth child born to my father and my mother's first. Seventeen years separated my parents' ages. My father was European born and my mother was first generation American, born in New York.

My memories from the infant stage of development to becoming a toddler are very slight. I was told by my parents numerous times at age three that I was chief controller of the local park sandbox. I demanded that each child there make their mudpies to my size specifications. My parents had even taken pictures at the park with their brownie box camera to show me in later years.

When I turned five, my brother arrived in May of 1945, when World War II was coming to an end. My sister, seven years my junior, was born in 1947, and the last in the birth order was my youngest sister, born in 1949. This sister was born with grand mal epilepsy and profound mental retardation. This had to be the beginning of the end for my family which, up until then, had portrayed the "Leave It To Beaver" scenario. The family really began to disintegrate bit by bit not long afterward.

Doctors and close relatives, including my very controlling father, begged and pleaded with my mother to place my sister in a special home or institution. They did not want her to live with us on a day to day basis. My mother would not hear of it; not even after the neurologist sternly urged her with the same advice. He strongly admonished her not to jeopardize the mental and emotional welfare of the remaining three siblings. I was nine years old, standing there in the doctor's office, listening to all that was being said. I will always remember that very dark day in my life. It had repercussions for decades to come for me and my siblings.

How right that doctor was! Things took a path of dysfunction that reaped havoc for all concerned. Two of us experienced emotional breakdowns, requiring long-term care. My brother was first at about 18 years of age. He had numerous electric convulsive shock treatments. He was a very sick young adult. I fell into a mid-life crisis at 51 years of age. I needed years of therapy and long-term medications for deep clinical depression. The shock of breaking down, feeling like Humpty Dumpty, broken into a million pieces, motivated a journey that began six years ago to find my wellness and wholeness and soul healing. As for my middle sister, she escaped the worst of it. However, she did experience many years of anxiety.

Living with a retarded sister, who had multiple seizures for a good part of the day, was hard for us all. It was difficult for any of us to invite a friend or two to our house and especially no one of the opposite sex! My father emotionally left the marriage and thc family early on. He began to barrage us with his shaming behaviors and things went from bad to worse at our house. All three of us seemed to withdraw inside ourselves, frightened to speak our feelings or even cry! I felt my parents' silent messages and the disease was beginning to take its stronghold in our family system.

To protect myself, in the best way I knew how, I became very active in local Girl Scouting activities. It was my outlet for personal survival. Outwardly, I was seen as a as a smiley, outgoing and happy child, but I felt as though I was dying on the inside. Inwardly, I felt abandoned, unloved and very empty. I was gaining weight, obsessing on high calorie foods and filling up inside with overeating. I was to remain that way until six years ago, and, it was then, back in 1991, that I hit an emotional bottom and began to seek treatment.

FEELING THE URGE TO FIND HELP

As with many school teachers, I had the summers off. It was finally time to acknowledge the deep sadness that I was beginning to feel day after day. Still, not being too conscious of what I was really doing, I found myself sitting opposite a female psychiatrist, on a very hot summer's day in Miami, and not truly understanding how I had gotten myself there. What on earth was I to say to this Freudian therapist, who sat there in silence? I saw her twice that summer and each time I sat there mumbling and asking something about what kind of experience menopause was going to be. It was becoming more and more obvious to me that I did not want to be there. I made no further appointments with her.

However, I worked with a male therapist for a year and a half. after that summer experience. I was still spinning my wheels and going nowhere. I had learned to speak in a little more than a whisper by that time. This therapist assured me that he came from a happy and functional home. I finally realized that I did not need to be there either; that probably he could not empathize with me and my deep woundedness and emotional pain. By this time, I was in the midst of constant clinical depression. I experienced classic symptoms: remaining in bed for a good part of the day, crying and crying, anxiety and panic attacks with severe spiraling and shaking with frozen fear. I felt as though I was in the middle of a huge tornado! So, once again, I set out on a journey to find a more appropriate therapist.

The third time, I struck gold. My dear friend, Rena, seeing how very depressed I was each day and getting worse, literally took me by the hand and escorted me to a Wednesday night group for Adult Children of Dysfunctional Families, led by my present therapist. She requested that I attend for three weeks in a row and then if I did not feel that it was for me, I could go elsewhere. Well, that never happened! The first fifteen minutes that I spent there that first evening told me that I was very much in the most perfect place to begin my journey back to wholeness and wellness. Little did I realize at the time, but a Higher Power, much greater than myself, had opened the most beautiful door for my healing.

OPENING UP TO HEAL

My therapist, Don Moore, a John Bradshaw trained professional, began to take me under his wing in early 1991. Very, very slowly, I began to hear his gentle and kind words and to my surprise he was listening to me very intently. As a result, I began to open up and share. I felt like I was dreaming it all! It was amazing not to be shamed and blamed for my feelings and behaviors! I had permission to cry and begin to feel my anger inside and I did!!

I have filled buckets and buckets with tears in the past six years in his office. I not only found my anger, but a host of deep fears that I have held in and repressed all my life since I was five years of age. I was learning to trust for the first time in my life; to let go and share all that was on my mind, my heart and my soul for so very long. I had found one of the most highly qualified professionals in the mental health field to help me, and I knew how very blessed I was.

This book is dedicated to Don Moore, L.C.S.W., for whom I hold the highest regard and respect. He is my mentor, guide, teacher and healer. Through his example, I began finding my way to inner peace. He is not only helping me to grow and mature, but he has helped me to find my own strong connection with my beautiful Inner Child, who became so stuck. When I light my Sabbath candles on Friday night, he is always included in my prayers.

For the first six months in therapy, I stared at the floor, barely able to say my name. I could not feel and I was very closed down. I was riding an emotional roller coaster. I was fighting to function at school in my role as a kindergarten teacher. Many days, I was not able to get out of bed or get dressed for work. At home and at school, I found myself hysterically crying out for help. I was pacing up and down the school hallways, talking to my therapist on my cellular phone. Many days at the beginning of my healing, my aide would be covering for me for a little while and I would sit in the back of the room doing her job!

I experienced a hard battle with breast cancer in 1993 that would have otherwise driven me to attempt suicide had I not been so well prepared with new recovering tools. I was beginning to attend Codependents' Anonymous meetings on a regular basis. I was fortunate to find a great sponsor named Ken. I was also beginning to learn to work the Twelve-Steps. About a year later I began journaling daily through all the tears and pain.

I was open to the healing. I learned more about John Bradshaw's work with codependency to better understand this disease within me. I was listening to many tapes including relaxation meditations, and lectures and books on tape of other renowned recovery speakers in the mental health field.

I invite you now to join my journey. Through my journaling for the past five years, I will share with you my experience on this the most spiritual path toward my finding my wholeness. Here we go!

"One can never consent to creep when one feels an impulse to soar."

Helen Keller

CHAPTER II

1992, Awareness and Challenge ... A Half Century Later

Starting from Scratch
Beginning to Journal
Traveling for Treatment
Medications

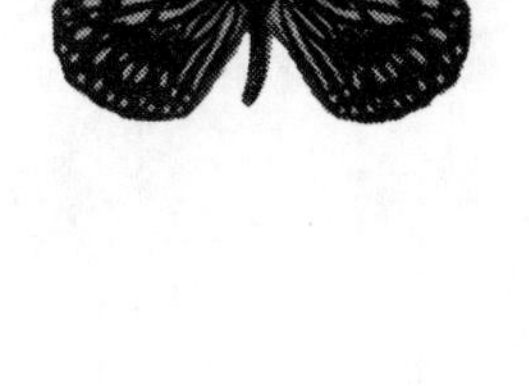

CHAPTER II

Although journaling is quite common, it is an excellent avenue for me to express my feelings on paper. Many a day in the past five years, when the tears came with all the depression, it was so cathartic for me to journal almost every day. Rereading all the entries that I have written and deciding which ones to select for these next five chapters, has brought me to a more intense appreciation of where I have been and where I have grown to today.

January, 1992

Dear Journal,

Today I decided to start my journal! There are so many issues that I am dealing with at once, I am in overwhelm. After one year in therapy with Don, I have finally started to open up just a little and share between my tears. No one has ever listened to me the way he does. His kind and gentle healing words are so foreign to my ears. He does not shame me and judge me like my family does. Since I was a young girl, I have always been told how fat I was. It hurts so much when they do that! Whenever I hear that word, "fat", I just want to run and hide and never come out.

I feel that overwhelming feeling of sadness and depression today. It is completely overtaking my mind and body with excruciating pain and anxiety. My spirit is all but gone. I think I want to give up and not fight, but I won't. I am where I need to be.

Dear Journal,

Today is the first day of the rest of my life and today I went hang gliding. I had to do something for surrender! This horrible fear that I have with doctors, all kinds of doctors, is so frightening, and just as a routine exam I need a sigmoidoscopy in the doctor's office! Boy, does Don have a job getting me ready for this one! I pray that he knows how to help me. I go next month in February. Help!!

Dear Journal,

Very early on in my recovery, I felt the need to find a good massage therapist. Many times this happens from feeling touch deprived. I found a jewel; his name is Robert Singer and he adds a beautiful dimension to my healing!

Dear Journal,

Today is the first day in months that I can truly say I feel some inner quiet. I am beginning to find my inner child that got stuck when I was nine, and the neurologist advised my mother not to keep my sick sister at home and she did. Today I feel more love around me than ever before. I am not alone; I have myself, my family, my Higher Power, my support team and my family of choice. Joy to my world!

Dear Journal,

So many things are beginning to happen. Don told me that I might need some help with medication to keep me more balanced. I am going to see a psychiatrist to help monitor an anti-depressant called Pamelor. Maybe something shifted in me last year when I was breaking down after losing 50 pounds. I am scared! I don't want medication. It has bad side effects!

February 1992

Dear Journal,

I was able to do some anger work at the Wednesday Night Group and again I am feeling so wonderful! The deep fear, shame and anger inside me sinks me down into that quicksand so many times! How did I ever get this wounded? I will find my way out if it takes every drop of energy that is inside me!!

Dear Journal,

Today I need to express a fear that I have also carried all my life; my fear of all medical procedures and anesthesia. Little Rachel is still as petrified as she was in that hospital operating room at five years of age! A dentist or even a barber in a white jacket brings out this fear!

Dear Journal,

I remember what happened to me when I was five. I had to have my tonsils out and the trauma of all that never left me. I can picture it as though it was yesterday. I can see me, right now, kicking and screaming like a maniac but to no avail. Three or four nurses held me down on the table and they put that horrible mask over my face to put me to sleep. I was so angry and frustrated when I woke up. They said I could have ice cream to soothe my throat, but I couldn't swallow anything for what seemed like a long, long time. I think my fear for doctors started back then!

Dear Journal,

Tomorrow I go for that sigmoidoscopy! Don has done so many meditations and therapy with me to help me relax and to let go. I can't relax, I am so scared!

Dear Journal,

It was horrible! I cried inside so no one could see. And that's not the worst news. They found a polyp in my colon and now I have to go to the hospital in April for a colonoscopy to take it out! G-d, why are these nightmare things happening to me? What did I do wrong?? I have to take these little pills two days ahead of time! I want so much to run away and not do any of this. Maybe G-d and Don will help me to find some courage inside!

Learning to trust trustworthy people is still so hard for me. I could never trust my father, when he was alive. He would disappoint me over and over again and never be there when he said he would. Right now, today, I cannot tolerate being disappointed. I am feeling unmanageable just thinking about it!

Dear Journal,

I feel the quicksand pulling me down today! I feel desperate to get out. G-d, I need your help here. The panic attack is so bad! I can't stop spiraling down. What am I feeling about myself? I feel like nobody. I can't be seen. I feel so ugly. I don't even want to go to my CODA meeting tonight. I just want to disappear. I am not here.

Dear Journal,

I cannot run away. I can work my first three steps. I can surrender this pain to my Higher Power (I think). I can talk to my therapist today and call my sponsor, Ken. I am so grateful that I have all these tools to help me. I have the use of this journal to help me to express my feelings too. I can say and write my Serenity Prayer. I can help myself a lot!

Dear Journal,

I was finally able to do some anger work in Don's office today. It felt so good! I didn't even know I had so much anger inside. I feel like a stronger person for having the courage to do it. I am discovering that I am very angry at my parents, my retarded sister and my brother who had a breakdown at age eighteen. Why did they have to get so sick? Maybe there's a lesson for me here but I just can't see it today!

March 1992

Dear Journal,

February is over and now it's March. I keep obsessing about the colonoscopy. I can't think of anything else! There's a big committee meeting going on right now in my head as I write about it here in my journal. Just five more weeks and I have to do this! Please G-d, I want no hospitals, no anesthesia and no colonoscopy! I am so depressed today!

Dear Journal,

My colonoscopy is just one month away! I must work on meditation and relaxations and visualizations. I have never allowed any doctor to give me anesthesia, not even when I had my children. I am petrified about all this!! I pray that I can handle it with all the help I have!!

Dear Journal,

I think that I'm beginning to better understand that when we are able to open our hearts and talk to G-d about all our pain, it can be easier to do the Third Step and let it go. Don is helping me at every session now through his wonderful meditations to allow G-d's healing light in to trust that I can be fine in any medical procedure. Thank G-d for all his talent and experience!

Dear Journal,

Today I am processing through my fear thinking and feeling more positively about this forthcoming medical procedure! I am learning that I can trust G-d and others and be okay. I am learning to trust my dentist and primary care doctors. I have trusted my therapist almost from the beginning. Today I am working on trusting the hospital team that will work on me. Having a Higher Power in my life today is the difference that makes the difference! Feeling closer to G-d gives me the permission to place my well-being with Him. In general too, I need to trust and have courage to walk through my fears in a healthier way. If I should fall apart in any way on that day, I will work to forgive myself; reminding me and Little Rachel that we are human!

Dear Journal,

I have been insatiably needy for attention all my life. That hasn't changed yet and I feel very sad about it. My house of origin was always so chaotic and there was never anyone to talk to about my problems. I always had to have what I wanted right then, with no chance to understand delayed gratification and experience it. For many years in my marriage, I was controlling and demanding my husband's attention so much of the time. I never gave him his own space, until the doors of recovery opened for me last year. So much shame is coming up for me today when I look at my sick behaviors from the past! I still cry about it.

Dear Journal,

Passover is coming real soon and I am not ready for all the work that this holiday demands. I am so tired from school, so stressed with this colonoscopy coming up real soon that I can barely focus and stay in the moment. I am still taking Pamelor every day and that only helps to slow the emotional roller coaster a little.

Dear Journal,

In the past I hid my pain in food. I am going to attend an OA meeting to see if I like the fellowship. I have so many things to heal from. It's like a laundry list. I want to work harder not to abuse myself. I have such a hard time accepting my body. I feel so ugly.

April, 1992

Dear Journal,

After a solid year of recovery, I have accomplished many wonderful things to keep me on a healthier path. A year ago, I was in a constant state of severe depression. Today I am beginning to feel the healing that recovery brings. The colonoscopy is just around the corner and although I am still scared, I will not run away. I will go and do the best I can. My husband and close friend, Perry, will be there for me. I have support from my Higher Power and from my recovery world down here on earth. Don has encouraged me so much. I feel safer.

Dear Journal,

Tomorrow is my big day at the hospital. I am scared, but I will take my fear, put it in my pocket and do it anyway! Releasing the fear will set me free!

Dear Journal,

I was awful! I don't know how I got through today! We drove to the surgery out-patient wing of the hospital at six thirty this morning. I did not want to go in! The two of them got me through the lobby and we filled out the last papers. I was crying. The very last moment before I went in, the doctor came out and told us that although he had promised me to let my husband be at my bedside during the procedure, he could not allow that today because of hospital policy.

I went crazy! I started to kick the chair and I was yelling at my doctor. I was about to go home when he said that my husband could stay with me for the first few minutes. I felt so betrayed! I would not take drugs to relax and I only let them do part of the procedure! I felt like I had failed! The doctor was pleased at least that he was able to remove the polyp. He said that despite this horrific fear that I still have inside me, I did alright! Don was very reassuring too. He said that I did it, I just did it my way. What an emotional experience!!

Dear Journal,

As usual, Don was so comforting. He didn't believe that I had failed. He reminded me of one particular affirmation in the meditations that he repeated to me over and over again that said, "Even if it's scary, I can be okay". I feel a little better about yesterday now. I did walk through my fear with the colonoscopy, even if it was my way!

Dear Journal,

I have gotten more in touch in my inner child, Little Rachel. I am getting to like me more and Little Rachel too. We have not had an easy time. Today I know that it is my job to reparent her back to health. I can do that. The adult me can nourish this little girl and help her to feel welcomed to this world!

Dear Journal,

Today I wrote my own healing meditation. I told myself many positive things. I told myself that healing is me mending my heart, mind and soul. I can pull out of panic and spiraling periods and recovery need not always feel like an emotional roller coaster. I am enough and I have always been enough! I was just never told that!

Dear Journal,

I feel the caring of my support team. This is the first time in my life, here in recovery, that I feel cared about and loved. It is just a miracle unfolding in my life. When the door to recovery opened for me last year, I did not know how to walk through the portal. The darkness of depression was very frightening at first. But, G-d and my support world were showing me the way. Now, I have numerous tools to always keep this door to wellness open. I am finding some answers. I am finding clarity.

May, 1992

Dear Journal,

I know that I am a codependent and in the process of healing. I hated the label at the very start and did not want it connected to my name, but then I realized that recovery is not an event, but a process. I feel that I can own some of my own power to be responsible for my behaviors and change what I need to change. I am perfectly imperfect and in the past I only wanted to be as perfect as possible. I allowed myself no room for error and I tortured myself when I could not accept me! I am learning not to be the people pleaser and the caretaker for the whole world too. I am growing. I feel it today.

Dear Journal,

Today I am exhausted from the ups and downs of this insidious disease, but after talking to my sponsor, Ken, and to Don, I was able to pull out of the depressing feelings and see things in a better perspective.

Dear Journal,

At our Wednesday night therapy group we do an exercise called, "Welcome to the World". Don does a meditation taking us back to the moment of birth and we welcome ourselves into this world with love, caring and bonding. I really do not feel that I was very welcomed to this world by my parents. By reparenting Little Rachel in this exercise, she can feel wanted and loved. This is a major part of my soul pain.

June, 1992

Dear Journal,

Today I allowed myself to completely unravel over feeling left. This feeling and separation anxiety comes up big time for me when I leave Miami or when others leave me too! I feel like the rug has been pulled out from under me and no one is there. Don is helping me through meditation to feel more connected wherever I may be to my recovering world.

Once I can feel this connection, I will be fine!

Dear Journal,

Today we are going to New York to visit our children and grandchildren and I feel shaky with a long weekend ahead. It's hard for me to leave my support area. Today I will pray and meditate that I have the strength to do this. I will work on staying in the moment and having a great time!

Dear Journal,

I have been feeling some severe hot flashes today. These are the first signs that I am starting to go through menopause. I can make this a devastating experience if I choose to. The tools of my recovery tell me differently. I can transcend the negative thoughts of aging and accommodate thoughts and feelings of how this can be yet another opportunity for loving me.

Dear Journal,

The sensations of my new insights are so healing. I can feel me beginning to walk the walk as I talk the talk. It is a beautiful difference from what was. I see it as my miracle unfolding right before my eyes! I am so grateful today for all the bounties and lessons that I am learning.

Dear Journal,

I still feel my woundedness and neediness today but, the pain is lessening as I connect more and more with my Higher Power and His energy. The G-d of my understanding, understands me and when I relinquish control, life flows more easily. Then and only then can I feel a measure of inner peace, serenity and tranquility that I seek. I am coming into my own awareness.

July, 1992

Dear Journal,

I have been feeling pretty well but I know that these periods of wellness are sometimes short lived. I need to be vigilant with my behaviors to stay well. It is so easy to slip backwards. They tell me it's alright to go five steps forward and two steps back. I'm still not so sure of that. I am by no means the same person that started out on this journey eighteen months ago. Little Rachel was so repressed and frightened. Such is not the case today. Nothing happens in G-d's world by mistake. That is what my group friends tell me all the time. I want this last third of my life to be filled with beauty and peace and I am the only one that can accomplish all this. I cannot rush G-d!

Dear Journal,

I have insights now that I have never realized before. This "insight" is like a different vision. I know where I am going and whose coming with me. At first I did not know that Big Rachel and Little Rachel were embroiled in the battle of codependency. Today we are healing, right here in the precious present of life. Our journeys are in constant progress!

Dear Journal,

Don has been telling me about this great place where I can go to called Caron Foundation in Pennsylvania. I could attend for five and a half days. It is called, "Magic Mountain" because it had been a monastery and still very much a healing place. I came home from my session today, anxious to discuss the possibility of going there. It sounds wonderful!

Dear Journal,

My husband thought Caron was a wonderful idea to do more intensive work on my recovery. I am going to make reservations to go in August. One friend from my CODA group, Barbara, has been there too. I will ask her some questions after the meeting tonight.

August, 1992

Dear Journal,

I ordered tickets for my trip. I am getting a little excited but, on the other hand, I do not want to leave my support area for so long. I have this anxiety with separation but I will get through it! Don is excited for me too. He knows that this will be a good thing for me and Little Rachel to experience. I leave next week!

Dear Journal,

I feel so nervous just packing my suitcase! First, I take a jet to Philadelphia and then I fly on a nineteen seater propeller prop commuter plane to Reading. Caron is just thirteen miles outside of Reading in a little town called Wernersville. I leave in just two more days. Gulp!

Dear Journal,

Here I am on the plane, by myself (and with my Higher Power) and feeling pretty shaky. I don't know where I will be having dinner tonight and with whom. I have so many unanswered questions. I have such mixed emotions about doing this! I can't forget that G-d is right beside me!

Dear Journal,

The plane just landed at the Reading Airport. It is so small for an airport. The van is waiting to take us to Caron, but I am not ready to go! I 'm scared. I will call Don's answering service and just leave a message. I need to hear a familiar voice from so far away!

Dear Journal,

Wow, is this a big place and so beautifully nestled in the mountains! Caron sits atop a low mountain peak and that's why they call it Magic Mountain. I hope that some of that magic will rub off on me this week.

Dear Journal,

As we all walked in the door to register, they took Polaroid pictures for our files. I am feeling so tired and drained from the trip. I just want to take a nap but no time for that. We will be taken to our rooms soon to unpack and get ready for dinner in the dining hall.

Dear Journal,

Dinner was scary. All those new faces and no one to talk to yet! In a few minutes we go into our first introductory session. Maybe things will get better. Tomorrow we begin group therapy!

Dear Journal,

We stay in our group of ten for everything we do here. There are two therapists that will spend the week with us. I am working to stay open and not closed up. I want this to work for me and so I know that I must do the work in a little while. I will meet everyone in my group.

Dear Journal,

This work is hard! We are doing anger work and family sculptures of our families of dysfunction. I hope they don't do mine! The tears just flowed watching others do their work. The two therapists are very nice and attentive to us all. I feel a drop more comfortable now than in the beginning.

Dear Journal,

Tonight I felt I was in crisis! This most wonderful therapist, Glen G., who had done some sessions with us, sat with me for over an hour and helped me through it. The work and the horror of the past were right here in my heart and my mind. Glen was so supportive, like a Don of the North!

Dear Journal,

Today we go home. It's been a spectacular experience being here. The people in my group are wonderful, finding their way on their path to wholeness, as I am. I don't look forward to the plane trip home but I am happy to go back to Miami. I miss my husband and my support groups very much! I will miss the professionals and the clients I got to know here this week!

Dear Journal,

I can't wait to share this wonderful experience at Caron with my groups. Barbara, from the Wednesday Night Group, went to Caron a few years ago and treasures the experience too! This was a big step for me!

September, 1992

Dear Journal,

It is no surprise to me today that I chose teaching as my career choice. Many of the professions are attractive to codependents because they are caretaking career opportunities. I have learned many valuable tools of recovery during the past two years. Many times I use them wisely. Sometimes I falter and that is okay. I am always grateful for my Higher Power, the Twelve-Step fellowships and my professional support system.

Dear Journal,

Today I am feeling sad about starting school! I love my work in kindergarten but it is so hard to focus on it when I go in and out of crisis feelings! I will do the best I can under the circumstances.

Dear Journal,

In two more days we will be celebrating the High Holy Day of Rosh Hashanah. This is the time of year when we go deep inside and look closer at ourselves to improve this one and only life that G-d has given us. This year, I am ready for the holidays with anticipation and awe! In ten more days, it will be Yom Kippur, the Day of Atonement.

Dear Journal,

Today I feel very excited! I am realizing more and more the changes I see in my behaviors compared to the old codependent ones before recovery. I am learning a most vital lesson in my life; I am learning that it's okay not to be okay. Some of the blockage that I had been experiencing came from not discovering that ten inches from my head down to my heart. This is what ultimately helped me to begin feeling my feelings. Working on daily affirmations will help me to feel the power of the words in my heart.

October, 1992

Dear Journal,

It feels so good! The self-esteem I never had before is rising. I feel it! A love I never felt before from others is surfacing too. The caring that I have needed from others for so long is abundantly here fore me now. For all this I feel humbled and eternally grateful; with all this, I am becoming the real me; the me I was always meant to be!

Dear Journal,

Today I don't feel so well. I must deal with my mother's angry feelings toward me. When I first broke down, two years ago, I tried to help her to understand what was happening for me emotionally but met with limited success. I invited her to a CODA meeting and she came and was okay. I introduced her to my sponsor, Ken. Soon after that, maybe a couple of months later, she began to express anger and feel even possibly guilty that all that had happened in the early years of my life, was her fault. I told her over and over again that that was not true at all. I wrote her letters to tell her I loved her and cared for her and explained my feelings about how her anger and rage at me was not helping me to get well. From there things went from bad to worse.

I had two emotionally absent parents and I am feeling the pain of that so much today! It is a terrible loss for me in this life!

Dear Journal,

With all my growth thus far on this journey, there are still issues where I feel very stuck. The more major ones right now are body image, holding on to control, emotional dependency feelings and neediness and sliding back into old behaviors. Today I am grateful that I can look at my "stuff" and still forge ahead to find wellness! My therapist and my groups make such a difference! So do I.

Dear Journal,

When I married at the age of 23, I was young, naive and so much in need of affection and loving care. After the honeymoon was over, and I had gotten an idea of what it was like to be showered with attention, the internal conflict began to surface.

All the dysfunction, all the depth of my emptiness from my family began to seethe inside and I was going into a multitude of shaky directions all at once. I was never feeling balanced or satisfied or secure or whole or happy. With my husband, I raised three children, by the grace of G-d. Although they are each codependent in their own way, they seem to function fairly well but my personal internal war is still raging.

I have had so much good fortune and still I carry so much pain! I want to feel whole and strong in the broken places. I chose this path of healing, when G-d opened the door wide and invited me to pass over the threshold! I am choosing to have a good recovery day! I realize that I can be resilient and buoyant on this awesome journey!

Dear Journal,

Recovery is an astounding challenge to really know ourselves down deep. I could never ask for what I needed or deserved before. I did not feel that anything had lasting meaning. My public self was doing its own dance and my private self was dying. My public self is how I survived for fifty years. I was somewhat obese and very sad! In the recent past it was difficult to accept my past behaviors, directed at my spouse and my three children. It devastated me! I felt so ugly, physically and emotionally. But slowly I began to emerge from the quagmire and now I am feeling a little more eager to become a more beautiful me. We all deserve to feel the wellness and the joy!

Dear Journal,

Today I feel Little Rachel in pain over her neediness to feel loved and wanted. I will do some work in therapy to help me through today. I have gotten a little stronger in my broken places but this neediness issue goes way back and I got stuck way down deep. I will be okay, I know I will!

November, 1992

Dear Journal,

Today begins a new month, time for Thanksgiving and also my birthday! Each year, on my birthday, I don't want the day to end. I feel so special on that day! I was born on Thanksgiving Day and several times in the past 50 years the holiday has landed on my birthdate!

Dear Journal,

Today felt like the hardest day of my life! I feel so devastated. I was on my way to a meeting tonight in the rain on Biscayne Boulevard when it happened. I made a turn onto the road when suddenly in the driving rain I saw a man dressed in white walk right in front of my car and I hit him! My feeling of panic was tremendous. His body hit the hood of my car very hard and then ricocheted about 50 feet onto the Boulevard landing face up. I got so crazy! I jumped out of my car and ran over to where he was lying and began to scream over and over again that I had killed him! The tears were streaming down my face like a waterfall!

I was just frozen with fear and guilt. A couple, who knew my husband and I from the Hebrew Academy, was driving past the accident and stopped to help me. The husband is a well known doctor from Miami Beach. I couldn't stop crying; I couldn't stop staring at the man bleeding profusely from his nose and mouth. He was covered in blood!

The doctor quickly called 911 for me and they came in a matter of a few minutes. The rescue driver told me that he would be okay; that he looked so awful because the nose and mouth are known to bleed that badly. It didn't console me. I was still hysterically crying. Someone called my husband to come down to the scene and he was so supportive. I will never forget this day as long as I live. Today is November 4, 1992!

Dear Journal,

Today I am still spiraling from my horrible accident last night. I called all my professional help and recovery friends. They all were so supportive. They calmed me down and helped me understand that I am human and I can make mistakes. It doesn't make much sense to me today but maybe I will listen to my tapes over and over to help me let go and forgive myself for hurting another person. I need to pray to my Higher Power now to make it through this nightmare!

Dear Journal,

I have so much support in recovery helping me after this accident. Thank G-d for all of it! I was given a citation Monday night and I have to attend traffic school soon. I can do that and be okay! There is a lesson here for me. I need to discovery what it is!

Dear Journal,

It is still hard to focus and function as well as I did before the accident. I am sharing about the accident at CODA meetings so that I can feel the horror of it fade. Next week I will go to traffic school.

Dear Journal,

Today is Thanksgiving Day and I am writing a poem of gratefulness and gratitude, for all my blessings, even the accident. I am so happy that the man I hit is okay! I am calling my poem, "Thoughts On A Thanksgiving Eve".

Dear Journal,

Today is my birthday and I am 53 years old. When I turned 50, I remember how devastated I felt to be a half a century old! This year I will work on feeling so fortunate that I have made it this far! I will not let it depress me in any way! I can do this!

Dear Journal,

Today I began traffic school. It is was interesting and a constant reminder to be more aware of everything that is going on around me as I drive my car. I never want to cause another accident! Never!

December, 1992

Dear Journal,

Today I wrote a letter to my therapist. Many times it is a good avenue for me to share issues with him that are hard to do otherwise. Today I needed to tell Don some of the areas where I still feel stuck. I feel so grateful just to have this life experience and I allow him to help me to heal on this journey! I must do the work!

Dear Journal,

This month my husband and I will be married 30 years! With what's happening in the world at large, people are amazed when a couple reaches three decades together and the relationship is getting stronger each day. We are so delighted in recovery to be having this opportunity to heal together after all the nightmare of dysfunction that we have both had in our lives until lately.

Dear Journal,

We have decided to have a party to celebrate. Most of our guests will be our close and supportive recovering friends and the little bit of family that we both have here in Florida. Our children and our five grandchildren from New York will be celebrating with us too. We are so excited! The party is in two weeks, just before Hanukkah and the holiday season!

Dear Journal,

Our anniversary party is just a few days away! We have gotten new outfits for the occasion. We have hired a photographer to take pictures and a four piece band for entertainment. It will be held at an excellent Kosher restaurant on Miami Beach. It feels so good that I can do all this in my healing process. I recall times, not so long ago, when an occasion like this was impossible to plan and have, being so depressed about life and living.

Dear Journal,

Everyone just went home. The party was so wonderful! I can feel the high I am on. Letting in the hugs and wishes of congratulations was a little easier this time around. I know today that I am really loved and cared about so much. All of this was so absent before my recovery door opened two years ago. It was a wonderful night. I will hold this experience in my heart for a long time to come.

Dear Journal,

The new year is right upon us; another opportunity to count my blessings and make a commitment to continue to walk the walk. Recovery is the best thing that has ever happened to my life aside from childbirth! I never plan to let it go from my life experience. I must continue to heal my soul and reparent my inner child, Little Rachel! I wish everyone a happy and healthy 1993!

"Courage is doing what you're afraid to do. There can be no courage unless you're scared."

Eddie Rickenbacker

Chapter III

1993, Active Recovery...
A Metamorphosis Begins

Reaching in for deeper feelings
Becoming a CHT
A second recovery: Breast cancer

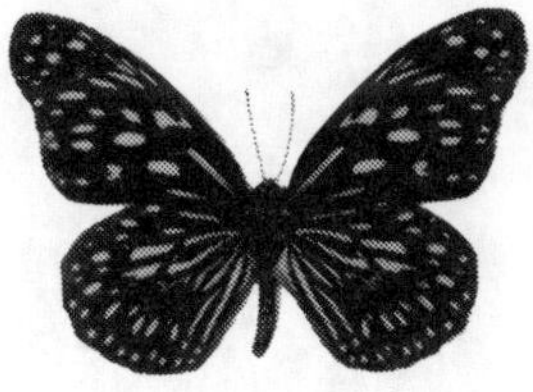

January, 1993

Dear Journal,

Today begins a new year; it is the first day of the rest of my life! Even with the roller coaster being very steep at times, 1992 has been a good year full of growth and wellness. It was so nice to spend this past weekend in New York with my daughter and son-in-law and our grandchildren. On this trip I did something really different; my son took me to my father's grave at a cemetery in New Jersey. This was my second experience there; I had gone in 1991. On the first visit, I went with a bag of dead flowers, my recorder and with the intention of giving him back all his shame and all the pain. I was living with him for so many years of my life! This time, I was a little more balanced and a drop more forgiving to the person called "father", who would never have been named, "Father Of The Year"!

Dear Journal,

I have just started to take the anti-depressant, Pamelor. I was asked a while back to just think about taking medication. I was told that it would give me some relief from panic attacks and severe spiraling and the deep feelings of depression that come over me more often than not. Sometimes, I feel so badly having to do this! The side effects seem so cruel but I must respect all my doctors' orders, if I trust in them to help me get well. Today I am thanking my Higher Power for leading me in all these healing directions.

Dear Journal,

Today I am writing a list of my feelings as this new year begins. All ten of them are positive, almost like a gratitude list. The one that just jumps out of the page at me talks about feeling the power of my own love for myself and for people that I hold dear on this journey! Hurray!

Dear Journal,

This journey, for sure, is not an easy one, but I would not exchange the opportunity to grow and become, with anyone or anything in this world! My scope of awareness and acceptance in the past two years has been wonderful. Healing and reparenting Little Rachel is how I can catch up and mature. My homework these days is to work the steps when I get stuck!

Dear Journal,

What a week this has been! It has been a week filled with much clarity; it has been a week filled with tears, pain and anger. It was a week where the definition of the word "boundary" took on a much healthier prospective for me for the future! I needed all these lessons with my issues.

Dear Journal,

Hard realities are difficult to accept, but they are our teachers. My expectations of others have led me to great feelings of disappointment. It is one of the hardest lessons that I am learning. Where there is no pain there is no gain is what I hear so often.

Dear Journal,

I am realizing more and more how much I love the butterfly and what it means to me. I feel my own metamorphosis happening right now! I must work hard to emerge from my own cocoon to become that beautiful butterfly that I love so very much. If other people do my work for me, to ease my way, I will never fly. This is the most important work that I will ever do in my life!!

Dear Journal,

I don't think that I realized until now how very devastated I have felt from my original abandonment issues! The strength of the disease and all the pain have given me this message of truth. I need to feel the freedom of wellness, the warmth of G-d's healing light, and the feeling of the wind on my face to win my battle with codependent disease, and, I will!. I do not have to feel such separation anxiety whenever I leave my support area or others leave for vacations, etc.

Dear Journal,

If the bottom line is acceptance with my core issues, I have a lot of work to do to overcome my compulsion with food. When I feel anxious or panicky that triggers it more than anything. Turning it over to my Higher Power works for me, until I take back my will! I can remember so clearly just two years ago when I lost 50 pounds. It was the most I have ever lost on a healthy food plan.

The change in my appearance was so striking, so different for me, that my mid-life crisis exploded right then. I have four or five closets in my home ranging from sizes ten all the way up to sixteen and eighteen. This yo-yo syndrome plays havoc for me on this journey to become healthier! So, here I am today with mountains of more awareness, a little thinner than my top weight and still puzzled and sad about it!

Dear Journal,

My mother was more than upset when I emotionally broke down two years ago. Aside from my retarded sister living with us for many years, my brother's breakdown came when he was about 18; it must have been all that she could take.

To protect herself emotionally, she found it easier to break ties with me and remain silent. Silent, she was and still is. She wants no part of me, her eldest daughter, and the pain from the neediness of wanting "mother" keeps me in tears whenever the word comes up from anywhere. I must work to detach with love from her everyday to rise above this! Then, there's the case of my deceased father. There is no closure yet. Working to psychologically detach from him also is a double challenge!

Dear Journal,

I feel very sad today with all this. I know that the more I can learn to be there for myself, the healthier I can feel. And I can be just fine without a mother's support, as sad as that is.

Dear Journal,

I know that I am finding my way. I have enrolled in a hypnotherapy course that will certify me to help others along the way too. I am so excited to take this giant step in the field and become a certified hypnotherapist (CHT)! Each year after this one, I must earn 15 CEU's to keep up my certification and be current.

February, 1993

Dear Journal,

Today I realized how angry I feel about so many things. I am angry that I am severely codependent; that I am shame-based and fear-based and so perfectionistic! I am angry that this disease could kill me if I don't work real hard to heal! I am angry at my parents and have been all my life. I am very angry that I have passed the codependency down to my three children and that my soul got so wounded! I am angry that I was abused emotionally!

Dear Journal,

Here I am two weeks later, I am still feeling the anger! I have worked on getting it out both at home and in therapy! I believe that the one thing that I am angriest about is that neither of my parents ever said that they loved me; I have felt so love starved and insatiable in my life and still do at times.

Dear Journal,

At this point in my recovery, I am not only grateful for my willingness to grow healthier, but I am very grateful for my spouse's desire to be there for me and for himself too!

Dear Journal,

Perhaps I am not letting go of all the depression yet. I cannot accept my mother not wanting me anymore! I truly don't want a relationship with her in her present toxic state. She might never again come back to me or even talk to me and I need to be okay with that, as hard as it might be.

Dear Journal,

Therapy has been such hard work! I cry a lot and many times work to defend my sick behaviors, even when I know that they are self-defeating. Another professional once told me that I do the best victim that she had ever seen! Boy, did that make me angry, however, today I am empowered to not remain in victim at all!

March, 1993

Dear Journal,

It is a miracle to witness how I have changed in the past two years! I can hardly recognize me! I always had to control people, places and things; it was my way or the highway. I have discovered that there is so much more to life than just surviving. This is a road to really feeling alive! The road is long and challenging and very rewarding! The road it lit by the healing light of my Higher Power and is filled with warmth and love. Life before recovery felt cold and lonely.

Now life has a new focus and dimension. There are times when I feel the challenge is too great and I want to run and hide. There are times when the unhealthy behaviors want to surface. But, the benefits of recovery are too great to ignore!

Dear Journal,

Today I had to look at my issue with transference with my therapist, even though it seemed too painful to voice. I believe that most clients or patients who come into one on one therapy and have been deeply wounded for so long, experience transference. For a time Don felt like my mother, my father, and grandparents all rolled into one!

Dear Journal,

I have started to go to a Reike Circle in a local crystal shop and the experience feels so good! Reike, I am told, is a universal healing energy that is delivered to the client using the Reike practitioner as a conduit for the connection. Reike is done one on one with appropriate touch to the body beginning at the crown of one's head. I am thinking about taking the next Reike seminar to become a Reike practitioner using this oriental ancient healing art!

Dear Journal,

In this new movie that just came out, "Scent of a Woman", Al Pacino, who played a blind ex-colonel, made such a profound statement that touched me so! He said, "There is no prosthesis for a soul that's been amputated"! Tears were streaming down my face, every bit of pain and emptiness that I had ever felt from the onset of recovery, just came rushing in. Is it possible that a person could imagine that their soul could feel so mortally wounded? I would like to believe that an amputated soul is just an illusion of a person's dire and outrageous pain. In healing on this journey, G-d is that prosthesis and bridge back to wholeness! I know that He is there for me!

Dear Journal,

I am beginning to give back to others, just a little! My sponsee, Claudette, affirmed me today by saying that people always look for me at the CODA meetings and our private therapy groups. It's still hard for me to accept that others care for me that much! I finally said to her, "Claudette, if you say so then it must be true", and I thanked her!

Dear Journal,

Each day I am working so hard to find all the courage I can muster up for a colonoscopy procedure that is coming up real soon. It's still at all the committee meetings in my head. Fifty three years and I still am so afraid of doctors and surgery. G-d, please help me to surrender this today!

Dear Journal,

Today I began to do the Twelve-Steps again with my CODA sponsor, Ken. He is a very spiritual man and is giving me wonderful guidance on this journey. It will take me quite a while to get through them. I am looking forward to doing a fifth step with him. We will sit and review the work I have done on the first four steps by sharing it with G-d and another human being!

Dear Journal,

My hynotherapy classes are going very well. In-between sessions, I am working with my friend, Phyllis, so that we can practice the inductions and the hynotherapy on each other!

Dear Journal,

It is still so hard for me to look at myself in the mirror because I still compulsively eat. I am practicing to say, "I love you" as I look into my eyes in the mirror and really mean it. Little Rachel goes in and out of the pain with her self-image. I have lots of work to do with her on this issue.

Today I want to tell her how much I love her skinny or overweight, all the time!

April, 1993

Dear Journal,

Today has been a kind of settling down day; settling down to the realization that I can be well and not remain addicted to the pain and the shame. I can play, laugh, enjoy a party or a good movie. I can let go of the depression that has not allowed me serenity nor peace for years! Opening my grasp and allowing G-d to be in control has been so hard for me and Little Rachel. It has been hard to fully trust. Today it is wonderful to just understand my past outlandish behaviors!

Dear Journal,

Tomorrow is my graduation from my hynotherapy training! I will receive my certification as a certified hynotherapist (CHT), through the National Guild of Hypnotists. During all our classes, we worked on each other, working through some of our issues using relaxation and visualization in a light trance called the Alpha state. This is one of the biggest pieces of professional growth that I can see in my recovery to date. I have this really glowing feeling inside!

Dear Journal,

April is coming to a close and although so many emotional healthy things are happening, I had a real scare this morning! I think I felt what might be a lump in my left breast. Talk about fright! What is going on with me now? My husband feels it too, but both my primary care physician and my gynecologist do not feel it upon examination. I feel better that the professionals do not feel what I do but I will keep vigil with it! What a day!

May, 1993

Dear Journal,

This weekend I will participate in becoming a Reike practitioner in Hollywood. Even if I don't use it, working with the circles I have found an art of healing that can benefit me alone or others along the way. Another beautiful door has opened for me to participate in another healing process.

Dear Journal,

My left breast still feels like something is not right. Every time I touch a certain spot, I can feel a bulge. It scares me to where I am obsessing on it a lot. My doctors say that I am fine. I guess, who am I to question?

Dear Journal,

This summer is the first time that my spouse will be going to camp alone in North Carolina to do his Judaism program and Bar and Bat Mitzvah lessons for the campers. We met each other at this camp and we worked there together for many years, so that our kids could enjoy the program. Two years ago when I began to fall apart, I knew that I could not work there anymore. Camp is such a busy place and I need my quiet.

This will be the first time in 30 years of marriage that we will be separated for two months. Right now, I am starting to dread being alone for so long. Actually, I don't want to be alone at all but he needs his space to experience what he enjoys doing so much. I hope that I will be okay. He leaves on Father's Day!

Dear Journal,

I have been on Zoloft now for the past month. This anti-depressant has some nasty side effects like losing libido and waking up in the morning with my throat parched as if I had been out on a desert.

Dear Journal,

Lucky me, John Bradshaw is coming to town soon and I will

be able to attend the weekend long seminar on codependency and shame, as an usher. I can't wait! I know that I will learn so much and grow too.

Dear Journal,

I am deeply hurting today. I went to my primary care physician for a yearly exam and wished afterwards that I hadn't. He shamed me badly about my weight that keeps yo-yoing up and down when the neediness and compulsivity with food strikes. He said that I was borderline obese and he wrote that in my medical file. That word wrenches my heart and mind and distresses me so! My family forever called me "fat"! I know that I need to exercise much more, have a balanced, lower calorie diet and continue to work in therapy and examine what is driving this addiction! And, believe it or not, this doctor could not feel any tumor in my left breast! The doctors can't seem to feel it. but I do!

Dear Journal,

This month we observe a two-day holiday called "Shavuot", which observes the giving of the Torah to Moses on Mt. Sinai. Holidays are still so hard for me. I feel uncomfortable many times not being able to go to my meetings or use the phone if I need to reach out for support.

June, 1993

Dear Journal,

Today this journey feels like a big roller coaster ride. Sometimes, I am so exhausted on this journey of pain and pleasure and I really want to throw the towel in and scrap it! Today I am angry that my care givers growing up were so sick and, in turn, I, as a care giving parent, passed the same emotional illness down to our three beautiful children! This is a very hard pill to swallow.

Dear Journal,

I received some disheartening news from my oldest daughter today. She told me that my two year old grandson might have a pretty serious problem. I saw it a little the last time I was up in New York visiting. I saw it in his stare and his glare. I saw it in his inability to react to most stimulation. I could see the possibility where he might turn inward and be lost. My daughter is hard at work to organize a special class with special teachers to work with two year olds that are exhibiting autistic symptoms! We are all praying that we can help him to come back to us!

Dear Journal,

I have side effects from the Zoloft. Just like the Pamelor,

Zoloft has uncomfortable side effects. Nausea, losing one's libido and experiencing everyday that dry, parched feeling in my throat. Sometimes I go to read a story to my class, and my tongue feels like it is stuck to the roof of my mouth! Sometimes I don't know what to do. I would like to not take any meds at all.

Dear Journal,

I feel so unsettled today; very burned out and very much looking forward to the end of the school year. I decided never to teach summer school again! I need this time off so badly!

Dear Journal,

In Ecclesiastes it says, "There's a time for every purpose under heaven." My time came about three years ago, when G-d touched me on the shoulder and led me to recovery's door. Recovery is such a challenging assignment! I have known that from the beginning, and there were several times when I just wanted out. There were times that were too painful and occasionally that is still true for me. There were days when I had trouble seeing the forest for the trees! Today I feel healthy enough, at times, to really tackle my therapeutic homework and do it well.

July, 1993

Dear Journal,

Each step of this journey today seems challenging, more joyful, and sometimes still painful. I am setting myself up for a disappointment when I have expectations for my behaviors to be better before their time. I feel so fortunate that I can come to groups and therapy and express my feelings openly and without fear. I know today that this is the very best gift that I have ever given myself.

Dear Journal,

Tomorrow morning I will leave to go to North Carolina to visit my husband at camp. I am excited that we will be together this weekend but, as usual, I feel the uncomfortable feelings of leaving my healing recovery area. I know that I can be fine this time!

Dear Journal,

The mountains are as beautiful as ever! This state has become our home away from home. We both worked to put our three children through the camp program. As a result, we became a real camping family for many years.

Dear Journal,

I am troubled knowing that my doctors still don't feel what I do in my breast. I am getting a little scared! It could be nothing or it could be something. I will have another set of mammograms taken again soon!

Dear Journal,

I am working on my fourth step with my sponsor, Ken. I must do a searching moral inventory of my whole life and then share it with another human being, which becomes the fifth step. It usually lasts for a good few hours. Ken and I are planning to do the fifth step next week.

Dear Journal,

Tonight my sponsor, Ken. and I sat for over three hours working on my fifth step. I am exhausted! I started with my whole life story to date and we talked about my character defects and other ways that I can grow in my recovering process. This is the first time in my life that I am beginning to feel a genuine sense of some wellness. I feel a healing straight down to my soul. For the longest time, the soul wound felt so huge and resounded with so much pain. Things are changing!

August, 1993

Dear Journal,

Parents! What a distasteful word in my mouth! I am finally finding honest core anger with them and not keeping it so repressed, where it was for years! I could not feel the impact living with a dictator father and a very passive aggressive mother!

Dear Journal,

It feels really warm and nurturing to have my husband home after being away working at camp for two months. We talked for hours, catching up on what's been happening in our lives for the past eight weeks. It was a challenging experience for me this summer to be alone and enjoy my aloneness. I know now that I can also thrive as well as survive.

Dear Journal,

Today I am not feeling that well emotionally. What a funky space to be in when the new school year is just around the corner. I need every ounce of energy and talent to handle it all!

Dear Journal,

School begins in four days, right after Labor Day. I am feeling very tired and limp at times with little enthusiasm. Yesterday I started to feel strange in my left breast. It does not feel like pain. As soon as I can, I am going to make an appointment for another mammogram. I have been so concerned about this since last April. It's time I start screaming a little if no one can feel what I feel in my breast! It's been there for five months!

September, 1993

Dear Journal,

School is very stressful, not like when I began 30 years ago! The roller coaster ride is very painful. It gets better but it doesn't stop. I can't stand to feel insatiably needy; I can't stand to be shamed! I feel ill, feeling so fat! The word "ugly" comes to mind immediately. I don't care what others think about me; I want to be pretty for me! I have a gut feeling that this next mammogram will be bad news! I am scared! It feels better to release some of this pent up anger, even on paper!

Dear Journal,

I was right! The mammogram showed a fairly large tumor

in my upper left breast! My mammogram tech, Judy Sorge, to whom I have been going yearly for the past five or six years, was at first surprised to see me back so soon since April. She told me that she could lose her job if she said anything about my films. I was freaking out and asked her several times to tell me something!

The only words that Judy could say to me, and not get into trouble were that if they were her films, she would go to a breast surgeon for an opinion! That's all I needed to hear! I cried all the way home from that office, not having a clue to where to find a good breast surgeon! In my tears, I felt me saying, "G-d, please give me a chance to really live before I die"!

October, 1993

Dear Journal,

My friend, Jacque, suggested I call a surgeon in Miami Shores, who she said she liked. So, frantically and holding my husband's hand so tightly, I made the appointment for tomorrow afternoon, after school. Thank G-d this is happening after the mid-life crisis and not before. I could never handle any of this without the tools I have acquired from the program.

Dear Journal,

The doctor was not warm or friendly. He saw how hysterical I was. I told him about my clinical depression and my horrific fear with medical procedures. He said he just wanted to examine me; that he never did needle biopsies at the first appointment. I could see from his face as he was examining me that he would do the procedure anyhow.

Through my tears, sheer terror was streaming through my body. I felt like I was going to die tomorrow! My husband held my hand as I lay stretched out on the table. The tears just kept coming and coming. The doctor took three tissue samples and put them into a jar to preserve them for the lab. I just knew they didn't look good! Sometimes we just know. He said I would hear from him soon, in a few days.

Dear Journal,

Waiting for a biopsy report can drive one crazy! I waited for four days and did not hear a word. I was pacing the hallways at school, leaving my aide to do my job with my class. Pat was wonderful! Finally, I couldn't stand it anymore and I went into my principal and finally told her what was going on. She was furious that the doctor kept me waiting so long. Today was the fifth day. She suggested I call him right there in the office and demand the diagnosis from the lab. I did that.

I told him how angry I was waiting for the results. He told me what I already knew but he was very rude doing it. He said, "Mrs. Lieberman, your report came back showing a four centimeter lobular carcinoma malignant tumor." And, then quickly added, "And what makes you think that just because you are experiencing depression, that the lab is going to rush for you"! That's all I had to hear and I said, "I know one thing doctor; you will never, ever touch me again" and slammed down the phone right there in the school office. Everyone was applauding and affirming me for how I handled myself. I thanked them through all my tears and asked permission to go home.

Dear Journal,

I don't know which way to turn! I could go to my husband's school or call Don and ask for his help! I think I'll call Don and see if I can see him between appointments. I pray so!

Dear Journal,

Don said to come right up when I called him this afternoon. I could hardly see to drive. Cancer, I kept saying over and over and over! I do have cancer. It was cancer all the way and I want so much to live! Don was really wonderful! He gave me a hug and he prayed with me about it. He said, in a very gentle way, "I will help you in the best ways I know how to get you through this! You are not alone, you have your Higher Power, the program and all the support that we can all offer you in recovery." When I arrived home, my husband was there and we hugged for a long time on the living room couch, praying and talking, and even in my upset, I was grateful!

Dear Journal,

My mammogram tech, Judy, called tonight to see how I was doing and I fell apart. She was wonderful. Words cannot even explain it. She said that I was the first patient who she ever followed up on in all her years doing this work! I just knew Judy was going to be a soul friend to me! She said that she knew of a wonderful surgeon in South Miami who she used to work with and would go with me to see him!

Dear Journal,

My new friend, Judy Sorge, is so amazing! She came down with me and my husband today to meet Dr. "D", as everyone calls him. When we got way down south to his office, I saw his name on the directory. It read, Dr. Robert Derhagopian, fourth floor. "No wonder they call him Dr. "D", I said to myself.

The waiting room was packed with patients for both he and his wife, who share an office practice. Finally, they called us in. I was shaking and crying, both at the same time. We waited for about 15 minutes in the examining room. Then the door opened and a rather short, gray haired man walked in, in his long white coat with a very pleasant smile on his face. He said, "Hi, I'm Bob" and gave me a kiss on the cheek. I told him my name too.

I was in shock that anyone could be that nice to me, after the experience I had just had with the first surgeon. He acknowledged Judy, who was in the room with us and then examined my left breast and explained to all of us what was happening to me. I did have a good size tumor as the other doctor had said. He was very hopeful that I would be fine. He said lobular carcinoma grows very slowly and that I had been carrying it around for several years; that it blends in with breast tissue and is difficult to find on the films!

He also explained that I needed a lumpectomy to remove the tumor and to see if the margins were clean around that area. If they weren't, it would mean that I would need a mastectomy on that breast. We set the date for the lumpectomy for October 26! I left the office, feeling a little reassured, even though I was scared stiff!

Dear Journal,

My thoughts are everywhere. Living, dying, surgery, anesthesia, operating room and the word cancer circling around and around in my head. My most major fear in life had come true! I was so taken back that Dr. "D" was comforting and pleasant, similar to my therapist, Don. I have about three weeks to work with Don on meditation and therapy to help me get to the operating table, hopefully in better shape than I was in for the colonoscopy in April of 1992.

Dear Journal,

My life feels like I am in such turmoil! I think I want to leave school, probably take an early retirement. The stress at school has been wearing on me for years. This stress plus all I have to deal with on my journey is telling me that I might have a second chance to really live, if I leave teaching. I will go to see my principal tomorrow.

Dear Journal,

My principal, Trudy Edelman, was very empathetic and encouraged me to follow my gut feelings and leave the job stress behind. My friends on the faculty were also supportive and many affirmed me for having the foresight to take an early retirement. That's exactly what I plan to do!

Dear Journal,

I have breast cancer! I can accept that today. Last week I realized that I needed breast surgery, whether the tumor was malignant or not. So, I am beginning to look at ways where I can banish most of the deep fear from my mind, my body and my soul. Surgery and anesthesia have been major issues for me since I was five.

Dear Journal,

Today I did the most wonderful thing. I went to my dentist to help me relax and surrender to a very small amount of anesthesia. It was the first time I allowed anyone to put a mask on my face in 48 years! I am beginning to have more trust and can let go a little more easily than ever before. Wow!

Dear Journal,

I have a wonderful support person in my life, Jean-Claude Klein, Rabbi/Psychologist. He took me to my first Twelve-Step meeting! He has been helping me with the Twelve-Steps to work through all of this. Today he shared with me a translation from Hebrew to English that says, "G-d gives us the medicine before the disease". I found myself processing that all afternoon. His ongoing help never ceases to amaze me. And it happened exactly that way for me, the tools of recovery before the cancer diagnosis.

Dear Journal,

The lumpectomy is scheduled in eight days. Today I had to go for two hours of pre-op work at the hospital. I had blood work, X-rays and I signed release forms for anesthesia. I have been praying and meditating today to find my strength to face all this in a healthier way then I did the colonoscopy!

Dear Journal,

My greatest challenge today is to accept my responsibility to myself as I go through this surgery that is coming up in two days! I am nervous and also optimistic that I will be able to surrender my control to anesthesia and be okay. I am happy and ready to remove all the cancer cells form my body. My therapist, Don, gave me a mantra in meditation today that really helps. The words I need to keep close to me are, "Even though it's scary, I can be okay".

Dear Journal,

I know that I will work through this emotional pain and be fine. Time promotes healing and feeling my Higher Power at my side is giving me all faith to surrender. I remember so well prodding along painfully, surviving as a caterpillar. For the past three years the trek has become easier and easier. I am beginning to feel more and more like the most beautiful butterfly in the garden.

Dear Journal,

Today was one of the most remarkable days of my life. With my husband and friends, Perry, Carolyn and Judy, I was able to walk into the pre-op and get prepared for the lumpectomy. Dr. "D" was right there for me too. When I woke up, ten minutes after the surgery, Dr. "D" was at my bedside gently explaining to me that my tumor margins were not clear and that we would need to schedule the mastectomy soon. I did not go off the wall. I listened carefully and asked him if I can have the second surgery in three weeks. I said, "I need time to get emotionally ready". He said, "Fine".

November, 1993

Dear Journal,

Today I feel myself standing at a crossroads in my life and soon I must let go of an external body part that has been with me for 43 years. I am powerless. I have no choice if I want to have a chance to really live and be healthy! Life was a painful drag just a few years ago. I know today that existing is not living. I was stuck in the material here and now that seemed to compensate for all that lack of love and nurturing. I was so sorely missing it in my life up to that point. What I was doing and where I was going was all a mystery. Three years ago, my life began to move from dysfunction to the painful arena of rebirthing into an awareness that changed everything.

Dear Journal,

Losing a breast feels devastating at this moment! My sponsor, Ken, asked me how angry I think I am. I told him that I feel angry enough at times to destroy everything in sight, although I would not act on it. I have really been a hard working codependent this past three years, resistant to improving my behaviors at times, but genuinely present for the recovering process to work in my life.

Little Rachel has come from a shriveled, frightened and repressed space, to a maturing, growing and courageous inner child. I am so proud of her.

Dear Journal,

My husband and I are going to have some fun this week going horseback riding on a ranch in Davie. I am looking forward to that before the trip to the hospital. I am so grateful that my husband is so supportive of me and works to understand my turmoil in what's happening to me now!

Dear Journal,

Today I am working on visualizing myself without my left

breast. I have drawn it on paper to the best of my artistic ability, which is not too much better than stick figures. After my surgery, I want to help others through the Reach for Recovery Program to feel more comfortable. So far in my life I have walked through Hurricane Andrew to the center of the eye! Soon I will walk through the remainder of the storm and be just fine after my surgery!

Dear Journal,

Today I woke up feeling sad and depressed, almost like a mild catatonia. It feels like being suspended and immobilized. It's like a numbness and a loss of interest in the world. This emotional roller coaster ride is so troublesome for me. This is not where I choose to be and I refuse to allow myself to remain in this dismal space. I will work my steps and my program all day today!

Dear Journal,

I have two major insidious, cunning and baffling diseases, one emotional and one physical. Breast cancer is the physical challenge. I can feel stronger than the diseases. I can take loving care of myself and I will! I must take care of myself in the best way I now how.

Dear Journal,

I have decided definitely to take an early disability retirement from the school system. Eliminating this stress from my life will be wonderful!

Dear Journal,

Today I went horseback riding. It was scary. The horses were so far off the ground! The owner of the ranch said she would lead me around the paths and for that I was very grateful! As we rode together she shared with me that she had recently come through a mastectomy herself. That's just where I needed to be today, to hear some positive feedback!

Dear Journal,

Today I did a hypnotherapy session with a gentleman from CODA, who wished to stop smoking. He has just come back from Caron Foundation, where I had gone for help. Needless to say, I was not in the best space to do it but I allowed myself to switch gears and focus on the work I needed to do with him. I actively listened to his story, gave him good eye contact and a relaxation and meditation with an anchor to stop smoking. I will see him three or four more times.

Dear Journal,

Things usually seem worse than they actually are. Right now the surgery next Monday seems scary! Today I must say the mantra Don gave me over and over again, "Even though it's scary, I can be okay". Today I want to buy some modeling clay and sculpt what I will look like afterwards. I need to see it, feel it and be in touch with it. I need to fully accept what is going to happen to and for me.

Dear Journal.

Today my pain is screaming, "Please don't let them take my left breast away, G-d. It is my femininity, my source of sexual pleasure and it has been my friend for four decades"! This is one of the hardest things I have ever had to do! I know that a part of my body has gone bad. I must remember that I am not my breast or my disease!

Dear Journal,

My friend, Melanie Kaleky, who brought me into active recovery, is an operating room nurse. She has been so helpful today. She explained things to me that are easier to understand about the surgery. She is also helping me to better understand that losing the breast will not cause me to feel empty on the outside if I feel full on the inside. This is my constant battle, working to love myself inside and out!

Dear Journal,

I know that cancer cells are cells that are completely out of control! My emotional self was completely out of control three years ago. My surgery early tomorrow will help me to have another chance to balance myself and my life. I pray that I will be well!

Dear Journal,

Thank G-d that my therapist is so caring and understanding! He gave me permission to call him about 6 a.m. this morning. I cried and cried and he prayed with me and helped me to mouth the words of the Serenity Prayer. He gave me affirmations that I could be okay and helped me to find strength to walk into the pre-op once again with courage to see it through! When we arrived at the out-patient surgery building, I would not let go of the building itself! Boy, was I scared!

My dear friend, Judy, was with me once again, for support for me and my husband! What a gem! Finally they got me off the bricks and I slowly walked into the lobby, full of tears and fear. The nurses were so wonderful. Dr. "D" was right there encouraging me that everything will be okay.

The anesthetist came to my bedside to talk to me. I implored him to give me a few minutes before he put me to sleep to see where I was, and to show me the breathing tube that goes down my throat. He was so nice and allowed me that time to settle down. And then I felt more at peace with myself and with G-d and I allowed him to fully sedate me.

When I woke up an hour and a half later, there was Dr. "D" at my side with a big smile on his face! He was reassuring me that I most likely would not need radiation or chemotherapy, that the medication Tamoxifin would be all that I would have to take. I was so grateful to be alive and getting well from breast cancer!

Dear Journal,

I feel so good to be home again! I have two huge "hand grenade" drains to deal with, but that's the least of it all. My sister came to see me from the Mid-West. It was good to see her, especially now!

Dear Journal,

It is one day after my surgery and I feel wonderful! My sister and I are planning to go out to dinner tonight close by the house, hand grenades and all!

December, 1993

Dear Journal,

My friends were so happy and surprised to see me at tonight's Wednesday night meeting! It felt so wonderful to be there, better than ever before. I will have my drains removed in a few days. I feel so light and happy, happy even to see the tiny ants on the grounds and of course the butterflies in the air! I have never felt so grateful and so strong in my recovery! I am empowered!

Dear Journal,

I signed up with the Red Cross to take the Reach to Recovery course so that I could share with others my experience, strength and hope. It is such a wonderful way to give back some of the wonderful support that I have had with this experience especially!

Dear Journal,

I have begun to take Tamoxifin also known as Nolvadex. It is an anti-estrogen that retards new cancer cells from forming in the body. It has some nasty side-effects though, like so many other drugs. The worst one for me was gaining 35 pounds as the medication begins to work in my body. I have another chance to work on more acceptance with Don on losing the breast and body image issues. This is my next assignment and responsibility.

Dear Journal,

Last night in group I was just bursting to share about the pain of losing of my breast. I was in the safest place to share my ambivalent feelings with my close family of choice!

Dear Journal,

A brand new year is beginning real soon. My goals for 1994 are becoming very clear! This year I will continue to strive to remain in the moment and not project ahead or fall back into the past. This year I will work harder to observe and respect the boundaries of others and my own, especially with delayed gratification. I have discovered, added to everything else, that I have a disease of entitlement and expectation. I am learning that expectations can always lead to severe disappointment. I have had too much disappointment in my family of origin in the past. I want no more.

Dear Journal,

I am happy to be alive and well for this new year. I wish my family and close supportive friends and professionals a wonderful year, filled with physical, emotional and spiritual health for all in 1994!

"Every human being on this earth is born with a tragedy, and it isn't original sin. He's born with the tragedy that he has to grow up. A lot of people don't have the courage to do it."

Helen Hayes

Chapter IV

1994, Becoming the person I was meant to be

Healing my inner child
Becoming more honest
Working to surrender
Dealing with my Jekyll & Hyde

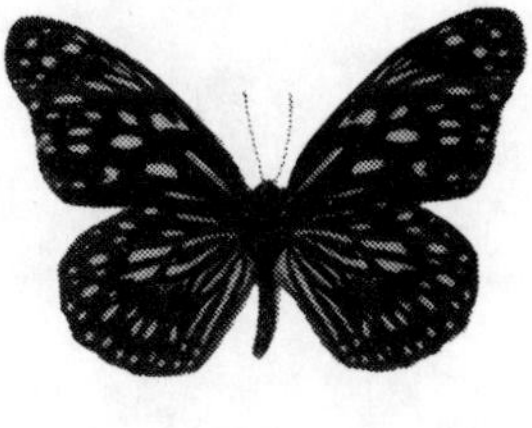

January, 1994

Dear Journal,

It is so good to feel alive and beginning a new year, but this post-op period from this most difficult surgery has left me feeling very grateful and depressed at the same time. I feel much more cognizant of how much I need a safe place to share all my pain and relief on this journey. Therapy has been an emotional life-line through all my core issues!

Dear Journal,

A real surprise for the new year came yesterday when my mother's doctor called me and asked me to go to her house and bring her to our local hospital. A cold streak went clear through my body. My first impulse was to just stay out of it. He told me that she was very sick and had not eaten for four days. I knew that I had to help her regardless of how intensely angry she is with me and my recovery. I admitted her to the emergency room and stayed at her side. I know how toxic she is for me today, but when she is down, she cries to me like a hurting puppy. The doctor told me he thought she has some kind of bowel blockage.

Dear Journal,

My mother was released from the hospital today and she

seems better. I will let her figure things out from here. She is too emotionally sick for me to be near her. I feel a little closed down today and not able to tap into any real feelings or issues. I feel really numb, really quiet and not able to cry or express any emotion.

Dear Journal,

Tonight I received my third medallion from Codependents Anonymous, from my sponsor, Ken. He spoke so beautifully about me in front of the group, sharing with everyone how far I have come in my recovery in the past three years. I cried listening to his words, knowing full well that I needed to take them into my heart and leave them there!

Dear Journal,

Through dear friends, Joan and Murray, I found my way to a wonderful and caring oncologist, Dr. Arthur Blaustein. He is giving me support just as Dr. "D" is, and finding that I can be just fine taking Tamoxifin and not needing radiation or chemotherapy. He says that my post-op blood work indicates a good prognosis that I can remain cancer free! I pray so!

Dear Journal,

I have feelings and thoughts about having a breast implant. I do not know all that it entails. I want to make some appointments with plastic surgeons to find out all I can. My dear friend, Judy, said that she would like to go with me, if possible. I am on a quest to see which way to go. Judy will be very supportive, I know.

February, 1994

Dear Journal,

We went to see a plastic surgeon on Miami Beach. He explained to us that a saline implant needs three or four stages to completion. It means at least three trips to the operating room! It might just all be too much for me. I'm not sure. At first, I felt so empty emotionally on this journey with my family of origin issues and now, after losing my left breast, I feel physically hollow and empty too!

Dear Journal,

Today I wrote a poem about losing a breast to cancer. I didn't realize that since all this began three years ago I have written several poems dealing with my recovery. Just another way to release my feelings and my joy and pain.

Dear Journal,

We are planning to move to Palm Beach County in a few months and I have mixed feelings about that too. There are so many friends to leave behind, friends that I speak to or see on a daily basis. I hope that when we do move in May, it will be a good transition.

Dear Journal,

Today is my youngest daughter's birthday. She is turning 22. I have been thinking how codependent a mother I have been to all three of my children!

Dear Journal,

I still feel out of sorts. I can't focus or settle into concentrating on any one thing for more than a few minutes. I feel sad and glad all in the same breath! Today I see my family doctor to talk to him about possible disability retirement from the school system.

Dear Journal,

I need to talk to my Higher Power that I call G-d. "G-d, it is so wonderful working on recovery from a disease that can make me feel so unmanageable. In each precious moment of life, I know today that You are walking by my side helping me to work through the problem issues all the way to the solution. I am surviving two very difficult recoveries and one very horrific past. I am in awe of Your majesty and Your wonders."

March, 1994

Dear Journal,

I need to assess what's happening in my life right now. I am working on a list of issues that really work well in my life and those that are not at this time. Just off the top of my head I can think of several positive things, like my Higher Power, healthier relationships, being cancer free, moving to the Palm Beach area, becoming an author, and all my efforts in therapy and recovery. On the other side of the coin, I am still dealing with codependent behaviors, accepting the loss of my left breast, detaching from a very toxic mother and continuing to work on a higher self-esteem.

Dear Journal,

I have learned so much in the past three turbulent years. I have learned to be a good listener. I have learned that I have some talent to help others with their pain too. I have learned that I have insight and that I can process with all my recovery tools. Becoming a certified hypnotherapist has opened new doors for me to participate in the mental health field.

Dear Journal,

Today is my son's birthday. He is 26 years old and doing so well professionally. He is managing a group home in New York for retarded adult males, as he works on his Ph.D. in psychology. We are so proud of him!

Dear Journal,

Today I must remember that no one ever promised me a rose garden, and if they did, it was filled with sharp thorns and stickers. I have learned to tend such a garden and keep away from the places that can hurt me. The roses are beautiful creations from G-d. They are created with such delicacy, such precision, such fragrance and such beauty! Nature never ceases to amaze me; the animals, the trees, the sky, and my most beautiful butterflies!

Dear Journal,

I have begun to participate in the "Reach for Recovery Program", sponsored by the American Red Cross. As part of a group, I am trained how to ease a woman's recovery following breast surgery. I am starting to visit patients either in the hospital or the home, teaching arm exercises and giving overall support. It was so wonderful when a representative from this program came to see me soon after my own mastectomy.

Dear Journal,

Three days following my surgery last November, my mother-in-law died right before my eyes. Her control and aggressive behavior toward me was even more powerful for me than the shame from my father. She, like my father, always told me how fat I was and how much weight I needed to lose! Today I have not gotten to forgiveness with either one of them. I hold a lot of anger with these issues!

Dear Journal,

I am still working on weighing the pros and cons of considering a breast implant. I have come up with more cons on my list than pros. When I am ready, I will find my internal answers with this. Right now, I cannot have closure with this painful issue!

Dear Journal,

Today is my mother's birthday. She is 76 years old, very angry and unhappy, sharp tongued and cruelly shaming! My choice is to remember that the doorknob is always on my side of the door. I cannot be with shaming and toxic people anymore!

April, 1994

Dear Journal,

I hate being overweight, no matter what's causing it, meds or food. I am pretty sure that there are not too many people that enjoy it! There are still many deep seated issues within. I have come miles in recovery. I have many more miles to go.

Dear Journal,

Today is a shaky day. My spouse was in our local bank during a robbery. People were in jeopardy. He was very frightened also. I will be happier when we move So will he.

Dear Journal,

Today so many positive thoughts and feelings are whirling around in my head and my heart. I need to include some of them today in my journaling:

Suiting up and showing up for the gift of life.
Remembering that I still have one healthy breast and my health!

Sharing warm close times with my spouse.
Buying a new home and having the freedom to decorate it.
Changing many old behaviors to new ones.
Finding the light at the end of the tunnel.

Enjoying my children and grandchildren.
Feeling grateful for therapeutic experiences.
Coming through two surgeries. Feeling the fear go!
Journaling my feelings. Sharing my story in poetry and prose. Finding time to pray, relax and meditate with serenity.

Dear Journal,

Today I was made aware of yet another possible side effect to my follow up with the cancer medication, Tamoxifin. Aside from the weight gain (35 lbs.), at the onset of taking the drug, dry mouth and loss of libido, etc., there is a higher risk for uterine cancer! Today I feel that if the disease doesn't get me outright, the medication to prevent it could. It's like the antidote could be more dangerous than the original disease of cancer. Just a few short months ago I watched my mother-in-law die of pancreatic cancer. It was just awful for me to watch her suffer! No matter how toxic she was in my life, it was so sad the way she had to die!

Dear Journal,

I am so powerless over my future, as we all are! We truly don't know what will happen for us even five or ten minutes from now. When I was diagnosed with a life threatening disease, I felt even more than powerless. I felt helpless that modern medicine might not be able to help me.

From all this thinking, I allowed and still allow myself to fall into depressive thoughts with the word "cancer". Many times, it seems, that the words cancer and AIDS carry the connotation of doom and disaster! I need to work on more affirmations with this disease, just as I do with codependent issues and low self-esteem. I can do that today!

Each day is a new beginning and I can work to let go of all this pain and suffering and from holding on to being a cancer patient instead of a cancer survivor!

I will work harder, as the CODA closing suggests, to concentrate more on what needs to be changed in me and my attitudes than what is going on in the world at large.

May, 1994

Dear Journal,

The process of this metamorphosis and change is a totally

amazing miracle for me. I was so very sick, so needy and frightened and in the wrong hands to find emotional wellness. With poor guidance, I very well could have withered away emotionally right then.

Today, in remission from cancer and most of the "insanity" of codependent disease, I have a wonderful chance to live, love and respect myself, to become the person that G-d has meant for me to be. It boggles my mind that I have the courage to take healthy risks and feel the faith in my Higher Power in place of the catastrophic fear that has dwelled inside me for so many decades! Today I feel that I am enough!

Dear Journal,

My therapist is away on vacation this week. I am learning the boundary of delayed gratification and the acceptance of separation anxiety. I am becoming aware more and more now that I might have a permanent chemical imbalance. Even with all the distressing side effects of meds, I must accept what I need to remain more balanced and healthy!

Dear Journal,

So much has changed during this past week. I am putting together the nicest and most comfortable house that I have ever had. A person's home is really his castle and the decision to move was a very good one for both my husband and myself! It is wonderful to be able to focus on doing "house" instead of "depression".

Dear Journal,

Very soon, in June, I will be reaching my half-year mark since the mastectomy. I will go to my new oncologist, Dr. Blaustein, for blood work to see how I am doing. I feel a drop scared and a lot excited!

Dear Journal,

My doctor, who monitors my medication, is weaning me off the Zoloft and beginning a new treatment plan for me with Serzone! Another challenge for me and my inner child!

Dear Journal,

Recovery is definitely a process; it is never an event! Recovery has brought more balance and stability to my life. Recovery is hearing a gentle, soft voice, guiding me forward, and much, much more!

June, 1994

Dear Journal,

My husband is getting ready to return to camp in North Carolina for eight weeks. I am so much better this year than I was last year about his leaving. I will go up for visitor's weekend and then again at the end of the second month.

Dear Journal,

Our youngest daughter is getting married later this year in October. Sometimes I begin to obsess on whether I will be alive and well for it! It's not so much that the word "cancer" scares me to death; I am not ready to die. I have just begun to live!

Dear Journal,

It can be very devastating living and being alone. I have learned on my journey that I can enjoy my aloneness and be just fine. This is my current issue, to ask for help when needed.

Dear Journal,

There is still a cold rational fear that I could die of cancer. I began to process this in my car today. I was overwhelmed with emotion. My car has become one of my sacred places. I can work through so much while driving. I can scream if I choose and laugh or cry too. No other person is there to hear me!

July, 1994

Dear Journal,

At this point in my recovery and in my life, I realize the importance of having an outlet to express my pain and my joy in complete privacy and confidentiality. This seems to surface as one of my biggest needs on this journey, to release emotionally!

After experiencing breast cancer, I have leaned that I can let go this underlying fear and retain my "sanity", but it is so hard right now to do this. My rational pain is saying, "Yes, no one is immortal, no one escapes death in our stages of human growth! However, I just began to find beauty and magnificence in my life. I felt that with a cancer history, my life could be greatly shortened! Please G-d, do not allow that to happen"!

Dear Journal,

Today I was sharing with my therapist, Don, that I believe the three most important words I said three years ago were,

"Please help me." That very short sentence set the wheels in motion for me by a power much greater than myself. It changed the remainder of my life forever! Doors swung open that boggled my imagination as a wounded inner child.

Dear Journal,

Here I am, a fairly simple earthling of my Higher Power's creation, looking for deep understanding on my way to acceptance. The insights keep coming and coming! Every human being is a walking volume of his or her own. It says in Ecclesiastes, "To everything there is a season and a time to every purpose under heaven." I do believe that! As my recovery began to unfold in therapy, with all my kicking and screaming and crying, I felt something special beginning to happen for me and it did big time!

Dear Journal,

I wrote another poem today entitled, "Starting to Dance". I have quite a number of pieces of poetic expression that have emerged so far for me on this journey! It feels good.

August, 1994

Dear Journal,

In one meditation my therapist asked me, "How can you love yourself less than G-d loves you?" I have so many things that I do love myself for, but my physical attributes are not too high on my list today. When my feelings are negative, I pull back into victim and I do not want to be there! I know that G-d must have his reasons for this lesson. Today, I am having difficulty understanding it after a surgery. I am thankful for all the inner beauty that I feel!

Dear Journal,

Today I am working on affirmations that will help me with my codependent disease. Journaling has become one of the best vehicles to process all my "stuff":

I am so much stronger in the broken places today.
I have keen insights to process issues now.
I can say "no" and "no thank you".
I am working hard to never accept shame from anyone!
I feel more whole today. The hole in my soul is closing!
I can ask for my needs to be met today, if possible.
I trust more.

Dear Journal,

I am visiting Vermont this week. My high school friend, Betty and I came to visit Vin Cundari, our English teacher and friend of 40 years! It feels so wonderful for the three of us to be together. As usual on this journey, when I am so emotionally moved, I write a poem. I have spent a good part of the afternoon creating a piece I call, "Present Alternatives . . . New Choices". They both shared that it sounds like my best one yet! I went to an evening Twelve-Step meeting and was asked to be the guest speaker. That was great!

Dear Journal,

Today I am feeling mild anxiety. I feel quite impatient, angry, slightly depressed and out of sorts. I cannot find my center. Today would have been the first day of the new school year that both my husband I will not be present for. Ultimately, we are both rather relieved that we are young retirees! The less stress, the better!

September, 1994

Dear Journal,

I am looking at my total program today. I asked myself the question, "How do I know that this program is working for me and my inner child? How do I know if I just didn't allow four years of recovery jargon to tranquilize me into believing it all?" The adult me feels that is a fair enough question after four years of investment time-wise, energy-wise and definitely financially-wise! As I began to process these questions, I realized that I am doubting my conscious sincerity to evolve and change my behaviors to healthier ones. Finally, I recognize the healthy and the light side of Rachel. I, too, must work to accept the shadow side. It has come time to deal with my Dr. Jekyll and Mr. Hyde!

Dear Journal,

Positive thoughts keep running through my mind today. At the very beginning of this journey, I was blinded by so many questions and so very few answers. Little did I know then how piece by piece and bit by bit the picture puzzle would slowly come together. Today, that original smoke screen is gone. I know that there is no perfection for man and what is, just is! When awareness was so new, how frightened I was of both living and dying. I was nowhere and I was everywhere. I was in a limbo.

Dear Journal,

I am beginning a training program to work on a crisis hotline. It looks like a challenging opportunity to learn about myself and to help others who call in. We will make referrals from computers. I have never made friends with a computer until now. It is an exciting time for me to give back a little of what has been given to me in recovery!

October, 1994

Dear Journal,

When it comes to forgiveness, it feels a little easier to get there with father than mother! It hurts to hear her spew her anger at me. It hurts to hear my mother say that recovery has ruined my life! On the contrary!

Nothing could be further from the truth for me. It hurts so much for anyone to be this angry and raging at me, when all I need and wanted was to let go of original abandonment and deprivation. I know that she is a very sick lady, who in her time did not have the opportunity or the permission to seek counseling or help of any kind. She had nowhere to go with her pain, except outwardly. And now, all this toxic energy is aimed at me for needing to change the family dynamics to get well!

Dear Journal,

This coming Sunday is a very special day in our youngest daughter's life. She will be getting married. My husband and I are so delighted for her and our future son-in-law. It is a time for our immediate family and our beautiful family of choice to celebrate and dance and rejoice together! That feels so good!

Dear Journal,

It feels so wonderful to say that I feel well, that I really know and understand today what peace is and what it is not. I have confidence in myself now that I can volunteer my services to others and make a small contribution to the mental health field! So many beautiful things are happening to me on this journey and I have a warm feeling that this is just the beginning! I have been a Coda sponsor for two group members so far. I'm beginning to feel so healthy!

Dear Journal,

One of my favorite recovery authors, Melody Beattie, at the close of her book, "Beyond Codependency", leaves her readers with such a special message. She says that if we surrender to the pain, we can then learn to surrender to the good. She says that it's there and more is on the way for us. She suggests to allow the love to flow to and from ourselves and no matter how good it can get, the best is yet to come! Today, I know how very important the word surrender is in my life!

November, 1994

Dear Journal,

I cannot speak for anyone else on this journey, only for myself. I was that very sick codependent who went to see a female psychiatrist four summers ago to try to talk! That visit began the most remarkable journey of my entire life. It was an experience that led me to find healing for my mind, my heart, my spirit and my soul!

At the beginning I had no spirit! I was drowning in a sea of depression, anxiety, panic and spiraling. The storm raged in me. It was my own personal Hurricane Andrew! There were several times when I wanted out, out of the pain of finding insatiable neediness, total emptiness and very hungry dogs in my "basement". I was minus any measure of self-esteem or self-love. I was full of self-doubt, distrust and co-dependent disease in every sense of the word.

Today, most of this is a memory of the longest tunnel that I ever walked through, from complete darkness into the healing light of my Higher Power. My salvation finally came when I began to hear and own the positive nurturing and gentle words in therapy. I am in a better space today. I am the "wind beneath" my own wings!

Dear Journal,

I am a very happy camper today. I have a spouse that is just getting in touch with his own emotional feelings for the first time. It is a real miracle for me to observe! He came from a family where the first time I walked into the house, I sensed the coolness and the strain of negativity. I felt the sickness in the house, but at that time I could not understand the dynamics of it at all!

Dear Journal,

Today, if the genie with the lamp came to me, as in the times of Aladdin, and gave me three wishes, these are what they might be:

1. My first wish would be to experience exactly what I have just recently recognized in my own life, the incredible feeling of what internal peace feels like. I would wish this for one and all.

2. My second wish would be for the energy of enlightenment to shower and embrace our very troubled planet, so that safety and more love could reign and not raging codependent disease!

3. My third wish would be that one day each week the world would stop what it was doing for two or three

minutes, repeat the Serenity Prayer, smell the roses and witness the moment we call life.

Dear Journal,

Probably I would be close to correct in saying that the metamorphosis of the butterfly is nature's most outstanding example of transition and change. It really is not a wonder to me anymore why I feel this close kinship to that process in my life.

Before the caterpillar beings its cycle, it is merely a round and plump many-legged insect, not too readily noticed in the scheme of things. But, once it begins to emerge from its cocoon and becomes more visible, it has taken on a beauty that is breathtaking to me. It is not a hardy or strong insect, but one of such fragile and symmetrical beauty, that it is awesome.

Dear Journal,

Today is a very special day for me! It is my birthday and one day before Thanksgiving and my first anniversary of remission from breast cancer. In this past year, G-d has helped me to understand that what I believed was the curse of cancer was a gift in disguise!!

December, 1994

Dear Journal,

Today was the first day in the past year that I wasn't in tears when I went to see Dr. "D", my breast surgeon! On past visits I was distressed, either about the surgeries or whether to have an implant, or just missing my breast so very much.

Dr. "D" said that I was looking very well and that I had a glow about me. He also said that I have a fairly good statistical chance of never having breast cancer in my remaining right breast. It was so good to see him! I feel that he is a jewel placed in my life and part of my ongoing support team. I will never forget how caring he was and so supportive on two of the most difficult days of my life!

Dear Journal,

Today is our 32nd wedding anniversary and getting better and better every day. What a recovering miracle for both of us to be working on ourselves, to grow and change and evolve together. It doesn't get much better than that!

Dear Journal,

Here I am at the end of another recovery year! This year has helped me to see how much the program and my Higher

Power are really there for me. I feel the longing to write a book about my experience, strength and hope. Perhaps, it will inspire another to find his or her own way to heal. I am so grateful for all that I am receiving on this journey. I pray that 1995 will be another healing year, working to find myself and my internal peace!

"Use your weaknesses; aspire to the strength."

Sir Lawrence Olivier

Chapter V

1995, The Journey to Wellness Continues

Patience, understanding and acceptance
Finding my inner beauty
Learning to let go
Dealing with my spouse's surgery

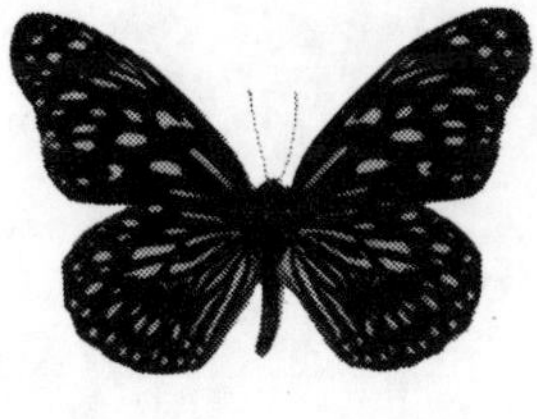

January, 1995

Dear Journal,

I had to write a poem today! It's New Year's Day and my husband and I went air ballooning for the first time in our lives with our good friends, Judy and Edward. It triggered me back to my hang gliding experience before the surgery! The first time it was for the feeling of surrender to my Higher Power. Today it was for the joy of floating in the grandeur of G-d's most beautiful sky, just beneath the clouds! What a wonderful way to begin this new year!

Dear Journal,

I am reminded over and over again of the recipe my therapist has shared with me to find peace. I call it my recipe to wellness. He says, "Patience will lead to understanding; understanding will get us to forgiveness and acceptance". It works for me in my life today, finally, finally, finally.

Dear Journal,

Sometimes this journey feels like an ongoing dream. In the past, I felt so hollow and empty, alone and unloved. Many times I felt unwanted and shamed and emotionally dead. However, that was not what all the darkness was about. It was about confusion and anger, envy and material possessions too. It was about feeling lost and stuck, fat, ugly and emotionally silent. It was about estranged parents, also empty and hollow and full of their own anger and disharmony. It was about no overt love or emotional nurturing, little understanding and no feeling of bonding for me and my inner child.

Sometimes, I don't know how I made it out to safety. Coming into the world of recovery, I was frightened out of my mind; no medical person could touch me and I was depressed and hurting more than words can convey. I did not know that G-d had plans for me to heal, some very special plans!

Dear Journal,

Today I am having thoughts of going back to school on a part time basis, hoping that I can focus on the material. I am so thirsting to learn. I will be happy for an Associate Degree in Human Services to compliment my Hypnotherapy Certification. First, I plan to take one psychology course and one chemical addictions course and see how that goes!

Dear Journal,

G-d opened yet another door for me today. I went to a local senior day center to observe how the professional facilitator led the group. I like working and helping the elderly. The facilitator had been there volunteering his services and was planning to leave. After the session, we spoke. He asked me if I would like to continue with the group after he left. I felt so overwhelmed at first and grateful for the opportunity to fill in for him! The center asked for my resume and I accepted the voluntary position feeling ready and confident that I could do this. I will begin in a few weeks. Wow!

February, 1995

Dear Journal,

Today I feel empowered, perhaps feeling a little like the person I was meant to be all along. I am learning that I can make a difference to others and I must always remember that I deserve that same random act of loving kindness for myself that I offer to others. I must also remember that I am no longer that human doing, but a human being taking life one step at a time!

Dear Journal,

Today I am writing about what I am observing in myself after four years in recovery. It is important for me to evaluate myself today:

1. I am experiencing many more days filled with serene

and peaceful moments than with depressive episodes.

2. I can focus better and remain in the moment more.

3. I know today that I do not need to play victim, I feel stronger and more confident to remain within my boundary decisions to be healthier.

4. A clarity about my responsibilities as a recovering person is more crystal clear now.

5. I will always need recovery in my life to feel my wellness, no matter what others think or say!

6. Acceptance is still difficult at times, but it is becoming easier to follow my program.

7. I feel the miracle of change within that began in the past four yeas.

8. I can talk about anything I need to discuss in therapy today, no matter how sensitive an issue it is.

And my list continues . . .

Dear Journal,

Two of our three children have birthdays this month. They

are two beautiful girls growing up with a better role model of mother than ever before in their lives! A blessing for all of us!

Dear Journal,

I wrote a great paper on "Depression in the Elderly" for school. Drs. Miles and Gardener are excellent professors. School has been wonderful too until this week. I have done very well on weekly quizzes, but now the mid-term is just around the corner and I am feeling the panic of not being able to handle studying so much material at once. Perhaps I might need to look at accepting that school might not be the way to go right now.

March, 1995

Dear Journal,

I have been my own worst enemy when it comes to having more acceptance with my body image. I need to remember that I am not my body. I am not my breast nor my weight. I will look in the mirror and work to see the beauty and light that radiates through me from my creator. My therapist does a beautiful meditation with me, when I stumble with this issue, called the magic mirror. In it, he works to help me visualize a projected image of myself that feels acceptable and comfortable to my consciousness.

Dear Journal,

I believe that my rite of passage is finding self-forgiveness. I can forgive myself for all the inappropriate behaviors of the past. I am not weak. I am strong enough to find my courage and use it, to find my inner-self, and the trust and love that has evolved within. I have caught the life preserver, I have found awareness beyond my wildest dreams in this lifetime already, and I have uncovered and discovered that I have a beautiful light side as well as my shadow side. All this is a miracle in its own right!

Running away takes effort too, but it keeps me suffering. Every time I come into therapy and share my deepest core pain, I relieve the suffering and heal the soul wound just a tad more. With recovery, life has taken on a new meaning and dimension so foreign to me in the past. I am finding myself spiritually, emotionally and intellectually. I am learning to give myself permission to keep healthy boundaries, and most of all to forgive myself and others who have hurt me. I can be perfectly imperfect and be just fine!

Dear Journal,

Today our son is 27 years old. In addition to running a group home in Brooklyn full-time, he is working to complete his Ph.D. in clinical psychology. Having a doctor in the family can be a wonderful adjustment to have to make!

Dear Journal,

School is not working out. Studying for the mid-terms is just much too much for me at this time. It would be best for me to leave soon, knowing that I have done the best I can and possibly try again another time. I will talk to my professors.

Before the end of class today, we all had an amazing surprise. One of the women in class, Kelly Phillips, walked in with an armful of books that she had just published! It was a book about eating disorders and her experience, strength and hope. It looks interesting! Maybe she will be able to give me some good pointers as I am mentally preparing to write my own book.

April, 1995

Dear Journal,

Today I facilitated my first support group at the senior center. Seven women came! For me it was an awesome experience, using so many skills with listening and empathizing when appropriate with my group members. This is an ongoing Wednesday morning group that I am looking forward to leading each week. I am grateful for the opportunity.

Dear Journal,

The power of this codependent disease is so deep and strong. When I was 32 years of age and feeling so hollow and empty, I was craving a fourth child to fill me up. I could never get enough! Fortunately for me, I did not act on this impulse! I could never have handled it.!

Dear Journal,

I have learned that I grow strength by strength, even when I take a step backward. I can now look back on last week and learn more about my codependency and grow from that. I am slowly learning to stop, look and listen to what the disease is saying and doing. My therapist, Don, many times tells me that he likes me, but not my codependent behaviors, when they come up. From this, I realized that I am not my behaviors.

Dear Journal,

In the past I would never believe that I could fight a good fight for my sanity. Today I do know that I matter and that sanity and serenity are so vital to my quality of life. I believe that G-d is happy for me that I am finding myself. I am jubilant too!

May, 1995

Dear Journal,

I want to move forward writing some of my book this summer. I have a message to share from all that I have experienced to date. I have a miracle to share too! It's still all in my head. I will begin my manuscript very soon.

Dear Journal,

Just as I feel with my other volunteer jobs, I feel comfortable facilitating at the Center for Group Counseling. Right now, I am working with young children in play therapy. As each session begins, it triggers me right back to my 20 years of teaching experience in the early elementary grades, working with five and six year olds.

Every Wednesday afternoon, I participate in a supervisory group meeting experience with from 40 to 50 professionals and facilitators present. It is an awesome meeting for me. I not only feel confident and comfortable there, I also participate in the sharing on occasions that come up. Our facilitator, Merrilee, is a very stimulating and experienced professional, who helps run the center.

Dear Journal,

Mother's Day brings with it many mixed emotions. With my children, I am working to become a healthier role model for them and for my grandchildren. However, the down side of the day for me is accepting that I have a mother who is not a mother at all. She wishes never to see me or hear my voice again, I've been told by family members. She is so very angry that she has locked the door and thrown away the key! Her repressed anger and guilt with her own life seemed to have exploded at me when I came into recovery and even more so after my mastectomy. I know that I am powerless with this issue and just need to detach with love and that is exactly what I am doing.

Dear Journal,

I am a year and a half after surgery and still toying with the idea of looking further into the pros and cons of going for a breast implant. I will see a few more surgeons, once again, and compare the risks to the benefits. This is still an open issue with me. I will find my way ultimately and come to a final resolve.

June, 1995

Dear Journal,

I have done a decent amount of homework on this issue of a breast implant and I am still at an impasse. Perhaps, it is because intellectually I understand it well, but emotionally is where I feel stuck. Is it wise to open my body up to possible infection? Do I need it so badly that I cannot be okay loving myself just the way I am now? What a loving message to give myself, loving me just the way I am!

Dear Journal,

When I began recovering, I had a gratitude list on my refrigerator as long as a laundry list. Sometimes I do not feel as grateful as at other times. Sometimes when my miracle is staring me in the face, I am unable to see it or appreciate it. My disease rejoices! I am not my disease, but it surely does a job on me whenever it wants to. This recovery is a major gift in my life and once in awhile my co-dependent behaviors signal me otherwise. I am learning better each day to handle it.

Dear Journal,

It's almost time for my husband to return to camp to do the work he loves so very much, working with children preparing for Bar and Bat Mitzvah. Each year at this time, I need to gather positive thoughts to remind myself that today I can enjoy my aloneness once again and be fine. Each year, I have the option to go and work there too, but I decline and need to stay home in my recovering world. This summer I will be just fine!

Dear Journal,

Today I am sorting and sifting through at least two thousand pages of journaling for my book. This is another commitment to myself that feels so good to keep; an experience that will allow me to share with others all the wonders of being a recovering person!

July, 1995

Dear Journal,

It's scary to feel this good. In the past nothing ever lasted and we all were waiting for the other shoe to drop. I can see and understand now exactly how much fear and fright I was living with all my life. I was depressed, scared, lonely, love-starved and touch deprived. If not for recovery, I would never have discovered and uncovered what really went on in my monumentally codependent family. Today, it is a blessing just to know that I wasn't totally out of my mind for no reason!

Dear Journal,

I am learning more and more each time I facilitate my senior support group! So many of our elderly have not found the path to inner quiet and peace and they struggle with fear and depression and the pain of coming to the end of their days. As I watch myself take steps to feeling more balanced and content, I see their willingness to brave the group and express their innermost thoughts and feelings. When I sense just the slightest bit of their own self-liberation, I can feel my own, big time!

Dear Journal,

Today is the Fourth of July and the date that my spouse and I met. It was at camp, the same one that we are still associated with. This December we will celebrate our 33rd wedding anniversary. When I sit down to process that a little more, I am more grateful than ever that our relationship has taken a turn for the better all the way around since recovery!

Dear Journal,

Today I sent my husband a love letter at camp. I have not done that for a very long time. It was a wonderful experience. In about three weeks I will fly to camp and we will drive home together. I am very excited.

August, 1995

Dear Journal,

The card that I received back from camp is probably the most beautiful and caring card that I have ever received from my husband.

What he said and the manner in which he said it was more than touching, so loving and so in tune with all that we have been doing in therapy and recovery these past years. All the pain of processing our issues together and working on our relationship has brought us to this beautiful place.

Dear Journal,

Expect the unexpected! That's what I have heard in the past. Today, when my husband called me from camp, his news was not good. He suffered a recent heart attack and has spent the last three days in the local hospital. Not wanting to upset me, he waited for his test results. He is coming home tomorrow for further testing. Damn!

Dear Journal,

Today my husband went for a stress test in the cardiologist's office. The results indicated a blockage in a major artery. Oh, G-d help him! The doctor has scheduled him to go into the hospital for an angiogram in a few days. Today I am praying that he will be well and not need any extreme procedures.

So many people care about us, genuinely care. It is such a good feeling to have so much support all around us! We are blessed and we will get through this one too.

Dear Journal,

After the angiogram today, my husband is scheduled for angioplasty tomorrow. Don sat with me in session and we prayed together that all should be well. He is so wonderful and supportive!

Dear Journal,

After a difficult angioplasty this morning, which necessitated placing two stents to open up the artery, the doctors were hopeful that this would eliminate the problem. If all is well, they said he could go home in a few days!

Dear Journal,

As I was coming up this morning to pick my husband up to return home, I was greeted with the news that he had just suffered a second heart attack. The doctors rushed him back into the operating room to perform another angiogram, which indicated the need for immediate by-pass surgery! I could no longer be strong and hold back the tears! It is so hard to watch all of this happening to my spouse! I love him so. Please G-d, bring him through this surgery safely!

There was no time to spare! I walked alongside his gurney and had but a few minutes to kiss him and reassure him that he would be just fine. His last words to me were, "Honey, pray for me", as they rolled him back to the operating room. My dear friend, Fran, stayed with me throughout the surgery. My friend, Judy, who was there for me for both my surgeries, was there too.

I was beside myself crying, pacing, sitting and calling Don for emotional support too. Today feels like I am having a nightmare. Thank G-d he is out of surgery now and resting comfortably in the CCU! I am sleeping here tonight in the surgical waiting room, so I can check on his progress throughout the night!

Dear Journal,

The pipe in his throat must remain there for about two days, until his body is stable enough to take it out! He looks scary and grey and unable to wake up yet! I have never felt so close to losing him as I did today! I pray that it is not his time to go! Our relationship has never been better; our feelings for each other never closer!!

Dear Journal,

Now, after three days of recuperating, he is beginning to show a very low hemoglobin, which could indicate internal bleeding. The doctors discovered a stress ulcer had developed and they had to do an endoscopy procedure in his room to stop the bleeding. G-d, hasn't he had enough? Healing from this will probably keep him here another week and that is fine. Here they can monitor him closely until he can come home and finish recovering.

Dear Journal,

Now as each day passes, my husband is becoming stronger and stronger. It will take time and patience for him to fully recover. So many people are wishing him well. Rabbi Brander and Rabbi Freedman came to visit. Our two older children and their spouses came down from New York to see their Dad. Our youngest daughter and our son-in-law, who live in South Florida, were right beside us all the way! Things are looking up for a healthier future, including more exercise and mostly a fat free diet!

Dear Journal,

My husband came home today! We are so grateful! Hurrah! Now I will have to don my nurses cap and help him all I can! I can do that with pleasure!

September, 1995

Dear Journal,

We went back to the cardiologist for the first check-up today and the report was very good. If all is well next month, we will plan a recovery party for everyone close to us to attend. What a happy day that will be!

Dear Journal,

I have learned that when a trauma or any other severe anxiety sets me off, I become very obsessive with food. This is where my disease kicks in and works to pull me down. I cannot allow this to happen to me again, and I will do my utmost to win this most difficult battle!

Dear Journal,

In a couple of weeks we will be observing the three High Holy days of Rosh Hashanah and Yom Kippur. This year the holidays will hold an even more significance for us, after all that has happened since early August!

Dear Journal,

We are beginning to prepare for the holidays by sending New Year greetings to family and friends. We are planning holiday meals for Rosh Hashanah with family and close friends too. Life feels good today! We are feeling the calm after the storm following a life-threatening surgery!

Dear Journal,

Today we are going shopping. It is a tradition to purchase holiday clothes for the New Year. We dip apples in honey for a sweet New Year and we say a special prayer over a new fruit to mark the beginning of the New Year. This will be the Hebrew year 5756. Yom Kippur occurs in about ten days from now.

October, 1995

Dear Journal,

This past weekend we had an incredible combination recovery and birthday party for my husband. The clubhouse in our development was filled with wall to wall family and friends. It was such a warm and loving experience for us. Everyone present was joyous to be there celebrating his good health!

Dear Journal,

Tomorrow, Yom Kippur, we dress in white clothing in the synagogue which represents purity as we ask forgiveness for the sins we committed against G-d. We do not wear leather shoes the entire day to show our humility before G-d. It is a very personal day of the year to communicate with our Maker in prayer. It is a fast day until sundown, when the Shofar or Ram's Horn is blown for the last time to signal the end of the holiday.

Dear Journal,

In a few days we are leaving for New York to visit our oldest daughter, who just delivered our fifth grandchild! It is still hard for me to go away but I can do this with less stress and discomfort now. It will be wonderful to spend some quality time with the family!

Dear Journal,

I have been really good to myself this week. I have felt more comfortable letting go, remaining in the moment and feeling more confident about it! My doctor is increasing my anti-depressants a little to help my chemical imbalance. It took quite a while to finally find the best recipe for me! I am very grateful!

November, 1995

Dear Journal,

I have "peeled away" many layers of the onion in therapy, touching and processing core issues during the past five years. I won't ever give up this good fight to be well and no longer be sick! I am very proud of myself and little Rachel for risking each step of the way and grow in maturity to better handle life on life's terms! My miracle of healing was my strength and courage to work for it. I feel that strength big time these days, as never before! I can honor myself by crawling out of the insanity of the past.

Dear Journal,

This month I celebrate my second anniversary being cancer-free! I couldn't be more pleased! Even though the side effects of the post-cancer medication are difficult to tolerate, like weight gain and intense thirst, I can do this and be fine. I have three years to go to stop the medication. That will be a day to just go out and dance in the streets!

Dear Journal,

Toward the end of this month I celebrate my 56th birthday and how overjoyed I feel to reach this occasion! How grateful I am to be alive and getting healthier all the time!

G-d has opened door after door for me, inviting me to pass through each one to grow stronger and stronger.

Dear Journal,

More and more I am getting to experience fun! I look for it everywhere! What a revelation in my life today!

December, 1995

Dear Journal,

Today I felt the inspiration to write another poem. I entitled it, "Recovering Magic". In it I talk about all the joy recovery means to me and the wonder of the whole experience. The two lines that seem to jump out at me say, "Slowly, ever so slowly the picture was crystal clear, that I was on a journey to live without the fear". To me, that says so much.

Dear Journal,

We just recently celebrated Thanksgiving, but every day is Thanksgiving for me these days. This whole recovering experience feels like a different language of understanding and a different level of just being. That I was able to see past the past and get to this day feels so liberating.

Dear Journal,

The holiday of Hanukkah is coming! It represents the story of the Macabee revolt for religious freedom. It is a fun holiday with dreidles and songs and eating delicious latkas (potato pancakes). This year I can enjoy it and focus so much better on what is happening in the here and now.

My husband and I were married on the second night of Hanukkah 33 years ago. This year as we light our Hanukkah menorah together for the eight nights, we have so much to be grateful for in our lives, especially for life itself!

Dear Journal,

Happy New Year to all! We are all blessed to be here beginning the New Year of 1996, and it's only four years away from the year 2000!

"The thing always happens that you really believe in; and a belief in a thing makes it happen."

Frank Lloyd Wright

Chapter VI

1996, Blossoming With Growth and Change

Getting a life
No turning back
Hospice
Off to press

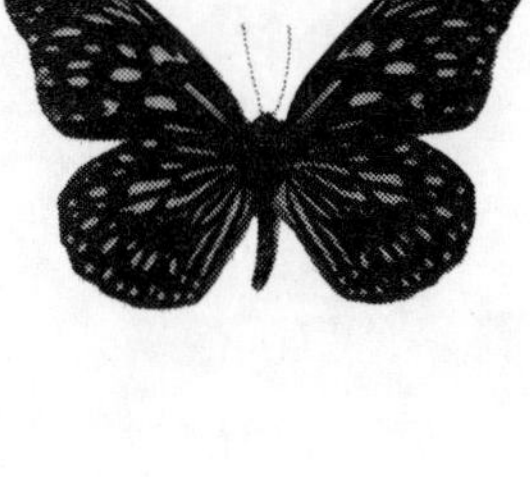

January, 1996

Dear Journal,

Good morning 1996! The beginning of a brand new year and more chances to grow and mature into that person I am meant to be! I feel so alive and well today! I feel that gift from G-d, as I continue writing my book and the words keep flowing out onto the pages.

Dear Journal,

Today I know that rational fear is the only healthy fear I need to deal with. My fear of G-d is the awe that I hold for Him. My fear of life and or death leaves me no life at all. That puts me back into emotional prison. It puts me back into the land of the lost! I have been fighting this good fight to be well ever since I began to feel my rebirthing. I feel the warmth and security of G-d in my life. Today I am loving and living more and fearing less!

Dear Journal,

If I allow irrational fear in, there is so much pain. Fear has stolen many years of my life when I could not let love in. It has put my intestines in knots and my head into a spin. Fear has driven me into seclusion to suffer. I fear what I don't know or understand. My fear blinds my eyes from finding the warmth that love brings. The face of fear does not allow me to love! On the other hand, love brings light into my soul. Love is life in its truest form. Love can bring nations together. Love is a very special gift to give others and to receive myself. I must respect both the love and fear.

February, 1996

Dear Journal,

I believe in myself today. I believe that I am here for a purpose, the purpose of healing and changing and evolving. I believe that I have more strength and willingness to outsmart my shadow side and remain in the realm of higher consciousness in thinking and behaving. I am not that sick codependent that began this journey just six years ago. I am working to become a beautiful butterfly right in my own garden!

Dear Journal,

Our two daughters have birthdays this week. Our oldest is 30 years old and the youngest of our three children is 24. It is wonderful to watch them grow and mature. Slowly, they are getting in touch with their feelings and being comfortable with a recovering mom.

Dear Journal,

The signs of serenity that come up for me are becoming easier to identify. I can focus on pleasant activities and really enjoy them. I can meditate and pray more readily and hear the inner quiet. There is no turning back for this codependent. I am on the journey to stay "weller" then ever before. The Serenity Prayer that I repeat each day holds immense meaning for me in my life now!

Dear Journal,

Today I learned that my spouse needs yet another surgical procedure, another hernia repair! The by-pass experience is still so fresh in our minds from just six months ago. This time I know that I can take this all in my stride and continue to be there for him. He was always fine accepting needed surgeries. I am getting better and better! He will schedule it very soon.

Dear Journal,

I have begun to study with a learned woman in my congregation to have a one time experience going to the Mikva. It is a traditional ritual bath that pre-menopausal married women attend every month to observe the laws of family purity. I was almost positive that I would be unable to do this at the age of 57, however I found out differently.

I am studying with Hindi Rubin. I need and want to do this for myself! It will be such a spiritual moment for me with G-d!

March, 1996

Dear Journal,

I am amazed every step of my way on this journey, whether I feel peace or the rage of the codependent disease! I feel that I am at a stage right now, working toward healthier independence. I see so much! I have learned so much and I have tons more to absorb and learn. This is a metamorphosis of more than just some behavioral changes. G-d is giving me a view of what it is like to be healing myself. Sometimes, I am so dazzled by all this!

Dear Journal,

Today I am looking at my attitude with gratitude. It has grown tremendously better since I put the first list on my refrigerator back in 1992. Today I am also writing a list of how I often sabotage my life so that I can become more aware and improve on these behaviors!

Dear Journal,

As March becomes April, there are so many wonderful

things happening! In April, we will be visiting our children for the Passover holidays and I will be experiencing the synagogue Mikva. I have all that and more time to work on my recovering issues and facilitate my support group!

April, 1996

Dear Journal,

I have watched me slowly, but surely, move from a life filled with negative dysfunctional behaviors to more positive healthy ones. I am so grateful that I am still young enough to initiate change in my life!

There was no beauty or peace in my life before recovery. Today I have more tears of joy than sadness and sorrow. After fifty years, I need to talk in therapy as badly as I need to breath! My life has real meaning and direction now. I know that I had to come through all the darkness to find G-d's light at the end of the tunnel. G-d tapped me on the shoulder six years ago and I responded. How wonderful!

Dear Journal,

Today is April 17. In two more days I will go to the Mikva. My dear friend, Shayna Batya, will be my "Shomerit" or guide and observer. I am thrilled and a drop nervous that I will make a mistake. I can be okay and correct things as I go. This week I am surely celebrating life to its fullest!

Dear Journal,

The Mikva experience was awesome! I felt at one with G-d in the warm ritual waters. I will never forget this opportunity that I had participating in this Mikva experience! Afterwards, Shayna and I went for coffee. I told her that I already had a poem in my heart and mind to put on paper when I got home!

Dear Journal,

Tomorrow we leave to go to our children in New York for the beginning of the Passover holidays. Getting together with family for the seders is always a joyous occasion. We will spend the last days of the holiday at home with close friends. Passover week is one of the most exhausting weeks of the year, with all the work that is involved with preparations but it is extremely rewarding!

May, 1996

Dear Journal,

We got some pretty great news today! My father in law, who loves to go on cruises, has invited us to go with him on a cruise to Alaska at the end of this month! At first the whole idea of being away from home base for ten days was upsetting. I will work with Don to release this separation anxiety to let go and enjoy this fabulous opportunity to see our 50th state.

Dear Journal,

Mother's Day is quickly approaching and that brings me such mixed emotions when "mother" is involved in any experience for me. My mother does not exist for me anymore. Her very sick display of anger and rage toward me has altered our relationship. However, I still have that original core feeling of needing "a mother" per say. Finally letting go of this pain will bring me more internal peace than I can imagine! Being the mother is a different story. Being acknowledged on this day by my children, is wonderful indeed!

Dear Journal,

We are getting ready for the cruise. This is our first one. My father and mother-in-law have been around the world three times! Everyone that has been to Alaska has told us it is an unforgettable experience. My father-in-law suffers with macular degeneration and is legally blind. He welcomes our company to help him get around the ship. That will be our pleasure.

Dear Journal,

It is May 28 and we are leaving today for the cruise. I feel a little shaky leaving but I will be fine. I will take all my recovering tools with me and work my program while there. I was also told that they have a Twelve-Step meeting on board the ship in the program each day. I hope so! I understand that Alaska is beautiful and the water is like glass!

June, 1996

Dear Journal,

Alaska is amazing! We have seen so many glaciers so far! We stopped at small seaports like Sitka and Ketchikan and Juneau is next. After Juneau we will go to Anchorage and then return to Seattle for the plane flight home!

Dear Journal,

What a trip! The ship felt like the most beautiful floating hotel! The two days of going and returning were very tiring and except for that it was just a great experience over all! In Anchorage, the last day of the cruise, we stayed at the Sheraton Hotel. where we arranged to get picked up by members of an OA group so that we could attend their meeting. After the meeting another member took us on a short tour around the city. They were very hospitable!

Dear Journal,

It's time for summer camp next week and this year my husband will only be away for one month. The doctors suggested that he stay for only four weeks after the heart surgery! Again, this year, I will need to enjoy my aloneness and have a good month. We will speak to each other almost every day and write some more letters. I will fly up when he is ready to leave and we will drive home together.

July, 1996

Dear Journal,

Today I wrote a letter to G-d. In it, I talked about some sadness that I have not felt now for at least six months. I wanted to put these feelings on tape this morning, however, time did not permit. I told G-d how often I ask for His help in prayer! Then I prayed for the courage and strength to surrender and turn over all the issues that I carry inside that cause me pain and suffering. I realized that I was doing my first three steps right in the moment.

Dear Journal,

This weekend I am attending a seminar at the Dominican

Retreat House. I am going with two other recovering friends. The theme for the weekend is self-esteem. I am so happy to have this opportunity to attend! I will bring my own Kosher food and eat with everyone in the dining hall. I always welcome the chance to work on my self-esteem, having had none for so much of my life until recovery.

Dear Journal,

The retreat was wonderful. We had group sessions with a psychotherapist and then broke down into smaller groups to personally discuss the topic. I asked to be placed on the mailing list so that I can know when other weekends are being offered on codependent issues.

Dear Journal,

I am leaving in a few days to fly up to camp and drive home with my spouse. We will stop in Atlanta to visit our very dear friends, Rae and Morris, and then come back to South Florida. Next month we are flying up to Long Island to attend our son and daughter-in-law's housewarming party. The whole northern family will be there!

August, 1996

Dear Journal,

Why do I feel today that I have been through the school of hard knocks and that I might always be a student at this institution? Life is so full of challenges, challenges and more challenges! My feelings are fragmented this week. On the one hand, I am totally up and very enthusiastic about working on my book. On the other hand, my heart is dragging on the floor with issues that are all my core pain!

I have wanted and needed to talk more this week than usual! I just want to scream out the anger that resides inside. I remember Tarzan and how he would let out the most awesome cry across the jungle. I guess that is the best metaphor and visual picture I can find to express how I am feeling!

Dear Journal,

The airport is a great place to people watch. Peoples' eyes talk to me. Either I see the joy of life sparkling from them or the deep sign of what looks like depression. For me, and many others, the eyes are the gateways to the soul! We are our own masters as to which path we will follow! The housewarming is this Sunday. It feels like it's going to be a wonderful trip!

Dear Journal,

Next month we will again celebrate the High Holy Days of Rosh Hashannah and Yom Kippur. We will go up north again for a family Bar Mitzvah. After the Bar Mitzvah, we will go to see my friend, Vin Cundari, who was my English teacher from eighth grade. This will be our second visit there. She has been an inspiration for me for the past 40 years! It's a very special friendship. We will arrive there in early October.

September, 1996

Dear Journal,

One of the few things that my mother told me before she threw me out of her life was that my father would promise to take us places time and again, and he rarely ever followed through. I believe this experience over and over again has made it so hard to accept delayed gratification when I need to wait for things to occur. After getting married in 1962, I took this behavior with me and expected things to happen and I could never tolerate the disappointment of postponements. I am willing to participate to heal on this journey. I have learned in the past six years, that I can still be okay even when things do not happen that were scheduled.

Dear Journal,

When I know my limitations, I can move ahead and heal! When I am judgmental, I am limited to sick thinking. When I am controlling, I am into very sick thinking too. When I am needing to be perfect, I have unrealistic expectations. When I am victim, perpetrator or rescuer, my behaviors are very codependent. Today, I am alive and more secure emotionally. I have sustained many losses, and I am okay. I need ongoing support and no one anywhere can lay guilt on me for having this need! I choose to be on this path today and every day that I have the privilege to be alive, alert, aware and accepting!

Dear Journal,

It is that time of the year again, after Rosh Hashannah, to celebrate Yom Kippur. On Yom Kippur we ask for repentance for our sins. On Rosh Hashannah, we are inscribed in G-d's Book of Lifc and on Yom Kippur it is sealed. I am sending our New Year cards to family and friends this week.

Dear Journal,

Today and in the past, I have inspired myself to work on my weight problem. I need so much help with this issue! Many times, I have felt how my body has let me down. It is still a little difficult for me to accept that I can be loved by others, even if I am not real thin or feel real pretty! I need to go one step at a time with this issue. So, the task at hand is to forgive me for thinking so poorly of myself. I was never told that I was pretty as a child. I was told how fat I looked over and over again a million times for decades. I internalized these shameful words in my head and heart. I am grateful that there are people in my recovering world today that love me just the way I am. I am beginning to feel that more and more. There is no turning back for me on this journey.

October, 1996

Dear Journal,

The Bar Mitzvah weekend in New Jersey was incredible, so much family together all in one place! We had such a wonderful experience there and we got to stay at a real mansion. The host and hostess were just lovely!

Dear Journal,

This is the second time that we are visiting here in Vermont. It is so beautiful and invigorating! The change of the fall leaves is so breathtaking. It has such a spiritual message for me. From the first moment I conceived the title of my book, I also visualized the book cover depicting autumn scenery.

I am feeling well today and able to remain in the moment and have fun with my good friend, Vin, and her roommate.

Dear Journal,

I have been a Hospice volunteer for a while now. Coming home was very painful! My good friend's mother who was my patient died while I was away. Last week, before I left, I almost knew that I would not see her again. I couldn't get myself to leave her bedside. I loved her!

Dear Journal,

So many roads can lead to our serenity. Surrendering to medical procedures of any kind is one remarkable step for me to get there. I have made a wonderful choice in my life today to work on one area of myself that I can change and plan to do that! For three full years the battle with what to do about a breast implant headed my list. Now, after long consideration and deliberation, I have decided to not touch that body area and be okay just the way I am.

I have decided to do mouth reconstruction. My dentist, Dr. Steven Goldberg, will remove all my sliver fillings and replace them with white bonded ones or crowns. He will make new veneers for my front teeth too. I want to cosmetically work on having the most beautiful smile that I can! It will make such a difference!

He is wonderfully patient with me and very understanding about where I have been with this issue regarding dentists for so long. I have shared with him how much I want to help myself and "change the things that I can change"! Going the dental route, I will not open myself to the possibility of infection, which is the one big risk for me with a breast implant. I feel so empowered to do this. I am just glowing!

November, 1996

Dear Journal,

Today my father-in-law gave us a second opportunity to go on a cruise. This time he would like to go to the western Carribean for a week toward the middle of this month. Again, I feel a little hesitant to leave and go away so soon! But, as before, I know that I will find the willingness to go and have fun when the time comes!

Dear Journal,

Yesterday I had a minor accident pulling out of my friend Rena's driveway. I am processing today that I felt too complacent. I was feeling so well that I was not focusing on what I was doing one hundred percent. This was another wake up call for me to stay on track.

Every day there are more and more lessons to learn. Today was the anniversary date of my big accident on Biscayne Boulevard on November 4, 1991! That night was so traumatic for me and I had additional big lessons to learn about being human. I needed to accept that I am and always will be just perfectly imperfect! Today I can believe that whole-heartedly!

Dear Journal,

My manuscript for my book is almost completed. I have been processing with my groups as to whether to put my picture on the cover or not. The downside of this issue is that I already have a raging mother and two siblings that are not crazy about me either. It seems not to be in their realm of understanding to realize the metamorphosis that I have made in recovery in the past six years. I have told my story in a very anonymous and protecting way! I decided I will put my picture on the cover! I will do it proudly. This is my time to share with others and I will publish in the early months of 1997!

Dear Journal,

Thanksgiving was so wonderful this year! My youngest daughter and son-in-law wanted to make the holiday for us in our home. My daughter and I got up very early this morning to make the turkey, stuffing and all the trimmings.

We enjoyed it all with our son-in-law's family and it was wonderful! I told them they set a wonderful precedent this year for many Thanksgivings to come!

December, 1996

Dear Journal,

It's hard to believe that this year is almost over! It feels like it has flown! Today I worked on my book for 14 hours! This is a first! I can focus so much better these days and months on the job at hand! I became so engrossed with what I was writing about, it was difficult to stop.

I have a wonderful person, Regina Moran, helping me to turn out the manuscript. She is very patient and a joy to work with! I have also found a terrific person named Dennis Beck, who runs Universal Graphics and Printing in North Palm Beach. He is a very patient and caring printer, who has taken me under his wing to help this novice author find her way. This was yet another wonderful door that opened for me on this journey!

Dear Journal,

Next week we have tickets to go with our close friends to see the Neil Diamond Concert that will take place at the Miami Arena in downtown Miami. I can't wait!

Dear Journal,

It took us about an hour and a half to wade through the heavy traffic to get to the arena! They delayed starting the show by half an hour! Finally we got into a parking lot and found our balcony seats. We had a surprisingly good view of the stage. For me, the concert was phenomenal! The songs were great. Only Neil Diamond could have sung them in his own inimitable way! We danced to the music all night!

Dear Journal,

Hannukah comes very early this year. Holidays too are becoming more fun for me to celebrate! My husband will, for the third year, light the candles at our Wednesday Night Group and tell the story of the holiday. I will make Latkas and applesauce for all to enjoy!

Dear Journal,

Next week we will celebrate our 34th anniversary. We have come so far together in our relationship, especially in the past six years. In the first few months of our marriage, after the honeymoon was over, our flaming codependent behaviors came into play. These attitudes were reflecting our family systems, which were both so sick! Today we are at a new level of respect and understanding with each other with tools that will always be there for us. Happy Anniversary to both of us!

Dear Journal,

This coming new year of 1997 has the potential to be a very exciting one! The book has a tentative date of publication about the middle of March! We will be editing it over and over again to find and correct grammatical errors. My friend, Arleen Baron, has agreed to edit the book with me. Thank you Arleen!

Dear Journal,

Our son and daughter-in-law will be coming down to visit us toward the end of January. We always love it when we can spend quality time together. We don't see them enough during the year, so close and yet so far!

Dear Journal,

As we plan to go to press in the next weeks, I am setting my sights toward scheduling book signings in the local bookstores, working on press releases and preparing for interviews with radio talk show hosts. My inner child is ready and so am I! Writing this book could be the beginning of a world of new experiences for me!

"A musician must make music, an artist must paint, a poet must write, if he is to be ultimately At peace with himself."

Abraham Maslow

FINDING MY CREATIVITY IN POETRY AND PROSE

CHAPTER VII

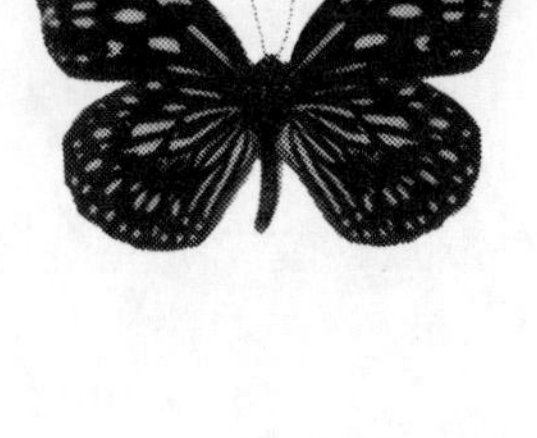

AN ESSAY IN METAPHOR

MAKING A PEARL

Once upon a time not so long ago, I was a very tight closed up clam, never dreaming there could be a pearl inside but a miracle occurred. On the way to that miracle, so much growth had to happen for me inside; I felt very much alone in this world and seemed to never care if I opened up at all. I was down at the floor of the ocean not able to hardly move. It was so hard to be alone down there and, at times, I just wanted to die away and become food for the many fish.

This metaphor of the locked up clam was me six years ago. I was stuck and cold and so depressed, I did not want to live. I obsessed about how much better the world would be without me. It seemed to make so much sense back then. But, in reality, it was not making any sense at all.

Who would ever have suspected that deep sadness and depression could become such a gift? Who would ever consider that I would use it as a major payoff to play victim for most of my life? When I blindly walked into the rooms, asking for some help, little did I know that the clam shells moved apart just a fraction of an inch. The pain was so great, the hopelessness and helplessness was alive and well in my sick mind; I could not take one more minute of this insanity. I was at my bottom!

Old timers in recovery rooms strongly suggested that I find a sponsor. I did what I was told and asked Ken if he would consider taking on the job. He graciously accepted the job and my life began at that moment to change for the better. I was led to an outstanding therapist and the pearl inside began to grow ever so slowly.

I discovered why I was so sad, so beaten and so depressed. I was quite angry. I began to work on my issues and safely worked to express the anger and the pain. I was not feeling so alone now. I was sensing that I had come home.

Now the pearl was the size of a garden pea and still evolving and growing. I found some answers that satisfied my heart, mind and soul. I couldn't always see the growth nor feel it, but that was coming too. The pearl was growing, more and more each day. It was becoming so beautiful!

And now after six years of ongoing recovery, I have grown so much that I can help others now in positive healthy ways. I can do my twelfth step!

I always keep in mind that I am human, that I matter, that I am beautiful inside and out and with this second chance to really "live" today, I will celebrate the occasion that I can live life on life's terms. My shell is fully open today and my pearl is so beautiful to behold. I hold that pearl inside me.

RECOVERY IS DISCOVERY

All of the dysfunction from my past,
Left an imprint deep inside,
And no one could deny,
That the hole in my soul,
Was opened wide;
Without a healing chance!

Deep pain and hurts,
Were constant reminders,
And the reality of it all,
Was my inner child running to hide,
To escape what she couldn't bear.

It happened slowly as can be,
A chance to grow and learn,
And see the beauty of recovery,
An answer to a special prayer.

I see G-d's light beaming through,
With every step I take!
I will never again feel all alone
With such healing underway!

The caring and love that's here
for me now,
From my family of choice is abundant,

It surrounds and warms every cell
of my being,
As my soul uncloses.

June, 1992

THOUGHTS ON A THANKSGIVING EVE

Thanksgiving eve brings thoughts of
gratitude for life and living ...
Day by day in a healthier way.
Thanksgiving eve brings thoughts of
universal love that's felt in channeling
our energies together ....

Thanksgiving eve brings thoughts of
appreciating family and our family of choice...
Day by day in a most loving way.

And Thanksgiving eve brings thoughts of
uncovering and discovering our miraculous
journey of recovery ...
Day by day in our Higher Power's way.

And so tonight on Thanksgiving eve,
as I reflect upon all of my blessings
I know that sharing our lives together

makes that beautiful difference ...
Day by day and week by week
in a most incredible way!
November, 1992

REACHING IN

Would anyone hold the pain that I feel,
just for a little while?
So that I could possibly catch a glimpse,
of what it feels like to smile?

Without the burden that weighs me down so,
without the shame and the hole,
letting go of the pain for a minute or two,
would lighten my sick heavy soul.

I dreamed I could soar like the monarchs on high,
and be free of it all till the end,
I dreamed that my Higher Power above,
is the one that can help me to mend.

And so I can give this pain to Him now,
for more than a minute or so!
I can give it to Him to hold now forever,
and find freedom by letting go.

Letting go of the anger and fear and the doubt,

and to learn to trust others too,
is a tall heavy order for me and my child,
when numbness was all that we knew.

I've mustered my strength and my courage too,
to reach in and pull the pain through,
no matter how hard this task is for me,
it's the best thing I'll ever do!

To finally feel well from this dastard disease,
to feel free and to let it all go,
to find peace in my soul for me and my child
is the answer to how we will grow!

August 12, 1993

THE CUNNING, CLEVER CULPRIT

A disease lurks within us,
working to strangle and sap our strength;
We're willing to fight back for sanity and peace;
Willing to go the extra twelve steps to freedom!

Yielding to help,
eye to eye, heart to heart and soul to soul.
Finding our way, discovering ourselves,
and the journey begins ...

Easing our pain, we find answers;
Soothing the soul, healing the hole,
Addressing the past, the shame and the guilt,
letting it go to a Higher Power.
Letting it go to grow!

Looking at today, not forward or back,
the precious present .... this very moment;
Healing days, caring friends, finding more answers.

Bringing in health, unlocking our chains.
The disease retreats ... we keep the guard.
We work the steps, we heal more wounds.

Blue skies, G-d's healing light,
love and warmth and safety,
and a monarch in flight.

FEBRUARY 25, 1994

STARTING TO DANCE

The movement, the tempo, it just wasn't there,
a glare of emptiness, a sad forlorn stare,
it lingered and hovered with tears, panic and pain,
in G-d's time, I kept hearing ...it gets better, the refrain.
A door opened to healing and much wellness too.
The dance started to move me, just slightly, but I knew,

that all wasn't lost, there was peace here on earth,
for me and my inner child...it was our rebirth!
The storm was horrific, dark, scary and long,
but today we both smile and burst forth with a song,
we worked hard to get here from the other side,
to sing and to dance and to no longer hide.
The gift of recovery is the dance that we do;
little Rachel and I are no longer so blue.
G-d's healing light now keeps us warm and safe,
our whole family of support does too;
We're all doing our dance of life together,
the most beautiful dance we can do!
The movement, the tempo, I feel it today,
a miracle to watch it unfold,
I am starting to dance, I am starting to heal,
I am starting to find my own way!

JULY, 1994

POETIC PROSE

PRESENT ALTERNATIVES -- NEW CHOICES

Sick beginnings....shame....pain....nowhere to turn....turmoil....swirling....spiraling....a hellish existence....and not really living.

Empty....alone....numbness....and about out of my mind....over eating....doing....and running away from myself....and the disease!
Needy, hungry for love ...
overworking....abandoned....repressed....angry....sadness and tears....still lost.
Total control....total darkness....cold....hollow and bleak days and nights....the child was so stuck....so wounded....so hurt....no escape....weight loss....and breakdown!
Then:
G-d....a ray of light....a path....Twelve-Steps....healing eyes....nurturing....caring times....tears of relief....and so much support!
Courage....less fear....some trust....more hope....time to heal....time to feel....new choices....bonded friends....finding my way....looking to me....recovering....relapsing....recovering.
Coda....massage....medication....meditation....therapy.... letting it in....hearing me....letting out the pain....accepting and forgiving....making amends....and letting go!
Tools....growth....challenge....change....chrysalis.... metamorphosis....the butterfly.
Then:
Cancer....breast tumor....surgery....mastectomy....No!
Finding my strength....reaching out....reaching in....prayer....using the tools....climbing the mountain....making it!

Breaking the cycle....healing the soul....so much gratitude....healthier attitude....loving life....loving me....the precious present....the child smiles....her eyes sparkle....much less shame....much less pain....no more quicksand....and no more blame.
Now:
We can sing....we can dance....and we can play....we can feel our feelings....we are finding our way....we are better today....we are okay....hurray....hurray!

AUGUST, 1994

LETTING GO TO MOTHER NATURE

A balloon in flight....a gondola....a breathtaking sight....drifting aloft....sailing on high....feeling the power of G-d.

Wrapped in the arms of Mother Nature....the silhouettes of her clouds form shapes and configurations challenging the imagination.

The landscape below....clear skies above....the roar of the gas burners....then the silence and serenity of just being.

Floating, freedom and the surrender of self to her gentle winds....shadows of the balloon against the majestic trees....reflections in the lakes below.

Soaring upward, slowly descending....landing....feeling the power of G-d....and the glow of feeling it all....being there....and experiencing the inner joy!

JANUARY, 1995

I'LL NEVER, EVER BE THE SAME

I'll never, ever, be the same,
but that's okay I heard me say.
I had to lose so I could win,
a battle that at first looked grim;
The cancer in my breast.

The psychic pain ran sharp and deep,
the tears came wrenching out;
My most horrific fear in life,
for me had come about.

I'll never, ever be the same,
and that's okay I heard me say.
I had to lose so I could win,
a battle that at first looked grim;
The cancer in my breast.

It's numb and very hollow,
this left side of my chest.
So I send love and light each day,

to that place that was my breast.

And although I'll never be the same,
yes, that's okay I hear me say;
I had to lose so I could win,
this battle that at first looked grim;
A cancer in my breast.

MARCH, 1995

THE MAGIC OF FEELING

It's gentle and caring,
the help here for me now,
at first I could not hear it,
at first I could not see how,

All the issues deep inside me,
were begging to come out,
I was so full of fear and shame,
I was so full of doubt.

I stood at a crossroad,
after stuffing so much pain,
so many times the silent screams,
resounded in my brain.

For fifty years I did not know,

just what to do, just where to go,
the choice was mine, the stage was set,
I took some risks, and challenges met.

It was time, G-d's time,
to find the real me,
not just the one,
I allowed everyone to see.
I began to feel and learn so much,
I began to search inside to get in touch,
with me and my child,
and the reality of it all,
the past and the present,
a true wake up call!

I have a teacher, a mentor,
helping to guide my way,
a soul healing person,
helping others everyday.

I have a Higher Power, a program
and support groups to attend,
a loving spouse, a family of choice,
and a wonderful chance to mend.

In five years time,
I have found that new me;
I can gaze into my mirror,

and love what I see.

I entitled this poem,
"The magic of feeling"'
That magic for me,
is to feel all the healing!

AUGUST, 1995

THE ALLEY

In a desolate and rainy alley one evening,
I thought I saw something peek out;
It had fiery eyes that spewed out danger,
and then just disappeared out of sight.

I wondered what it was lurking in the dark,
but, the storm worsened with thunder and lightning,
and for my safety, I headed right back home.

I tossed and turned in bed that whole night through,
it didn't leave my mind; Did it see me there?
Had I seen it before? Maybe I had felt it deep inside?

One question followed another, my curiosity
didn't subside,
and most of all I thought to myself, "What drew me there,
to that scary and unfriendly place?"

Maybe this disease type thing knew me,
better than I knew myself; Maybe I needed to go and
confront this mysterious thing in the dark?

I decided that night to return to the alley, as before,
and seek it out and discover the message it had for me.
I stood there anxiously in the alley, as quietly as can be,
hoping it would move about and discover my presence.

And lo and behold, there it was, standing in my range!
I slowly raised my rifle to get a better aim,
and then I did it, I wounded it, that part of me called
shame!!

OCTOBER, 1995

RECOVERING MAGIC

There's magic in the air for me, a special kind today;
By letting go and letting in, I'm finding a healthier way.

I never thought it was possible that I could change and
grow;
I never thought it was possible to know now what I know!

That healing takes community, love, trust and caring too;
That healing takes the courage to do what I must do.

I started at the bottom with quicksand everywhere;

I started processing all the hurt, who said that life was fair?

Slowly, ever so slowly the picture was crystal clear;
That I was on a journey to live without the fear!

Childhood days were so empty and I hungered for the love;
From mom and dad and siblings, but it was coming from above.

I have a Higher Power and a wonderful program too;
I have the best support team and feelings I never knew.

I feel a sense of peace now with the magic and discovery;
I feel the balance and the calm as I work on my recovery.

This journey is an ongoing choice and a commitment to repair my soul;
The wound is really closing now; There isn't a more wonderful goal!

I smile more today than ever; function and find my way;
I sing and dance and have fun now right here in the presence of today!

DECEMBER, 1995

THE SECRET

I have a secret deep within me,
Is what I am being told;
I feel the loss of childhood love;
It leaves me feeling ice cold!

I risked and shared my feelings,
That were erupting from every pore.
The neediness and the "insanity" from it,
Go deeply to my core.

I reach in for the secret,
So vital to discover;
For without it I truly believe
It could be difficult to recover!

From the longing in my heart and soul,
To fill the abyss with love and caring,
I feel so much pain with all this tonight,
But, what I hear is my honest sharing.

I have a secret deep within me,
Is what I am being told,
I will be so still; Patiently listen and wait,
For all G-d's answers to unfold.

"Rachel, your deepest fear and the secret within

Is plain enough to see,
Your battle with the horror is
That you might always be...
Never feeling satisfied
Never satiated with enough love,
Can you hear me when I tell you,
This secret comes to you from above?"

I own it now: I might always feel,
This original pain sensation;
To never have enough; To never feel fulfilled,
To be emeshed with such deprivation.
I had a secret deep within me,
no longer do I need to be told:
The pain of it all is subsiding,
Just one more miracle for me to behold!

January, 1996

MIRACLES

Lost and numb
Running away,
escaping to food,
no tools,
no support.
No insights and
no surrender.

Labile mood
more anxiety,
more panic attacks
more emotional downs.
Stabbing pain,
the rejection,
the shame
the fear;
All real and
core deep!

Dark shadows,
patterns of behaviors,
roots of control,
to strangle and smother.
An empty shell;
Alone, sad and depressed
abandoned and so needy.

Life seemed short
abrupt and ending.
Never content in
mother's womb.

A Greater Power
moved in the heavens
to acknowledge a Me!
A Me I could never see.

A beautiful side
ready to blossom.
Doors open
everywhere!

New tools, support,
insights,
filtering through
my fog!
Less labile mood,
less fear and shame,
and painful times
less severe.

My mind more open to see,
my heart more ready to feel
with help
love and trust,
surrender and peace.

Perfectly, imperfect,
finding my way
no more running to hide anger,
pain and fear.
I can cry today,
I can be okay, okay, okay!

February, 1996

CHANGES

G-d ignites
a spark in us all
at birth;
A blemish free
innocent
child.
No escaping
life's inflictions;
We sometimes
falter not
finding our
way.
The light within
diminishes
slowly.

So far down
we fight this
time of life.
Life rafts thrown;
Outstretched
arms
catch the ring.

The light
gets clearer,
step by step;

We find the love!

A spark
no longer;
flame,
tools,
change
a way of life.

Healing inside out,
letting go to surrender.

Finding the way,
forever a quest;
Forever
yearning for
peace.

That light within
burns bright ,
stronger and
stronger;
A Higher Power
leads the
way
to the
banquet table,
And I partake.

MY VERY SPECIAL PLACE

In the warmth of my home,
is a very special place,
a place where I feel G-d.

My spa, as warm as the womb;
It comforts and consoles,
and I am surrounded.

The azure blue sky,
is lined with crisp
white cotton clouds,
slowly drift before my eyes,
and there is peace.

The palm frons dance in
the wind and do their ballet,
and I feel free.

Free from the fears that
once drove me to eat and
hide all the pain inside;
Free from the agony of
living in the emotional
nightmare of family life.

As I lay in the water,

the sun shimmers through,
and falls on the Me
that I work so hard
to love...my outer
visible self.

This special place,
gives me time to reflect,
on the horrific past,
and all the beauty in the now.

I have climbed many mountains,
and the challenges were hard,
and as I worked, I grew;
And, still I fall back a little,
and that's okay.

I talk to my Maker and
I process my thoughts
and feelings about this one life;
The warmth of the water
warms my heart and my soul,
in this very, very special place.

April, 1996

HOLY WATERS - THE MIKVA B"H

I was first born
about five decades ago,
and then again last night;
The difference was awesome
this time...this time
I saw G-d's light!

A very special time
for a woman my age;
G-d opened the door,
for yet another page.
For a chance to touch
my Maker and see His
healing light too;
In a ritual immersion
that my Higher Power
brought me here to do.

This Jewish tradition,
is as old as mankind;
Brings spiritual connection,
to heart, soul and mind!
I am on a beautiful journey,
to find the essence of me;
I have worked so very hard,
and finally I see

That I am wholesome and
worthy and lovable too;
That I matter and have
evolved into a person...
brand new!

I have battled since birth,
to overcome so very much
in a family of dysfunction
that few could ever touch.
I feel so much better,
more balanced and content;
I am grateful and so happy,
for all that I've been sent!

April, 1996

I AM WHO I AM

I am who I am and
I'm not who I'm not!
Not the person who
couldn't feel at all
way back when;
nor, the deeply wounded
child of dysfunction,
suffering so, year
by year.

I'm not that little girl
waiting for that next
shoe to drop,
every minute of every
hour of everyday.
I am an emotional healing
person today.
Growing stronger all the time.
I have learned to travel inward
and look at my inner child,
to understand the pain and loss
so imprinted on her soul;

But with G-d's help and
total willingness,
my child and I are
finding our way to serenity
and peace, leaving much pain
behind.

Yes, today I am who I am,
and I'm not who I'm not,
I am real, content and beginning
to find a beautiful life in a
world of wellness and wholeness!

June, 1996

VERMONT

Vermont!
Autumn in the green mountains,
a breathtaking sight,
the hue on the branches,
swaying on high.

A palette of color,
and a time to reflect,
on this canvas of majesty,
a heavenly gift.
The dances of mother nature,
also messages from G-d aloft,
in clouds, streams and trees,
and the V-form of geese.
Vermont!

Trouble times left me blinded,
I could not see,
through the fog of my life,
until quite recently.

A struggle, a challenge
to be manacle free,
and to understand the disease,
I had to be me!

My sign is the butterfly,
all messages are clear,
transformation, spirituality in flight,
all help me each day,
to meet the challenges of my life!
Vermont!

October, 1996

THE MIGHTY POWER OF LOVE

At the moment of our conception
the gift of life begins
many have had the chance
of feeling and knowing
that mighty power of love.

Finally, oh yes, finally
the message came ringing clear
that I was among the fortunate
inviting love into my heart.

I feel the love inside me
at times, it glows so bright
I share it out to others
with understanding and insight,

I watch my mentor and my teacher

a message of continuous growth,
I'm becoming the person I was
meant to be
finding peace and serenity
inwardly.

There's magic in recovery
rebirthing and feeling anew
love is in the air we breathe
it is the essence of every
cell.

I am in love with the love
that's been offered to me
I walk now to a different
beat

Finding myself and being
myself
is the place I choose to
be.

At the moment of our
conception
the gift of life begins
many have had the
chance
of feeling and knowing

that mighty power of
love

Rachel Lieberman
February 13, 1997

" We ought to hear at least one little song every day, read a good poem, see a first-rate painting, and if possible speak a few sensible words."

Johann Wolfgang Von Goethe

CREATIVE CONTRIBUTIONS FROM MY RECOVERING WORLD

CHAPTER VIII

THE STAIRCASE

The staircase is marble and walnut,
the railings wind upward, spiraling.
Each step presents its own task
and difficulties.

No one climbs this staircase alone,
along the way hands reach out.
Sometimes pushing, sometimes pulling,
always upward.

Often, one tires on the climb,
occasionally a step, sometimes two
are taken backwards.
But then, if one has faith,
if fear can be overcome, the climb resumes.

Have you counted the marble steps?
Have you run your hand over
the walnut rail?
It's well worn by many hands.

Many have climbed before you,
many have turned back.
The staircase leads both up and down,
it's difficult knowing that
the pinnacle is never reached.

There is no perfection, only progress
 on this climb.
Doubt, selfishness, grandiosity and fear,
 these are the specters that line,
the way to the top.

But always, always,
 there are the steps.

The staircase is marble and walnut,
 the railings wind upward spiraling.
There are only twelve steps,
 each one represents it's own task and difficulties.

By: Don Moore

FAMILIES OF DYSFUNCTION

In the quiet of their solitude,
they each recall the pain.
The knowledge of their madness,
the dream that they are sane.

In the hallways of their sadness,
through corridors of despair.
Each time they look inside themselves,
they find that no one's there.

They are solitary prisoners,
locked inside their rooms.
Witnessing the hatred,
from their lonely silent tombs.

Each one to blame the other
in fear of their own shame.
Each one to call the other,
by his or her own name.

While lost in all their anger,
and captured by their rage.
The animals of the jungle,
lie trapped in their own cage.

By: Don Moore

RUPTURE OF THE SOUL

I feel it deep inside of me,
the empty aching hole.
The murder of my spirit,
the rupture of my soul.

I recall the very words,
from the moment of my birth.
You'll never amount to anything,
you have no human worth.

I struggle with my feelings,
then turn my face away.
My courage has eluded me,
on yet another day.

The mask conceals the anguish,
the rage can hide the pain.
My addiction keeps me warm at night,
when nothing can sustain.

Come break the bonds that hold,
then let us both be free.
To find the secret potion,
of things that cannot be.

I see it in my shadow,
when I've nowhere left to go,
I've asked life's questions honestly,
though I did not wish to know.

Each day's a celebration,
in the effort to survive.
If the flesh be only willing,
then the spirit stays alive.

By: Don Moore

CHRYSALIS

It happens every spring,
With the sun's relentless stare,
That the blossoms burst to flowers,
In the gently warming air.

And deep within a Chrysalis,
Where no prying eyes can see,
A butterfly feels the warmth,
And the yearning to be free.

But she's trapped in winter's ugliness,
That protected her from the cold,
And she has to struggle desperately,
so her beauty can unfold.

Then breaking from her Chrysalis,
On gossamer wings she flies,
On visions of red and gold,
She's lifting toward the skies.

The flowers nod approval,
As she gently flutters by,
That from such modest of beginnings,
She's now so pleasing to the eye.

Then on colorful wings of fancy,

She turns and flies away,
A Chrysalis no longer,
A butterfly she'll stay.

By: Don Moore

CHILD OF DREAMS

Once there was,
A child it seems.
Who spent his life,
Alone in dreams.

In a land of palaces,
And mansions fair,
No darkness existed,
When he was there.

But nothing's ever,
As it seems.
In a land of fantasy,
And of dreams.

And the lies that kept,
This land alive,
Crushed the life from all,
That could survive.

The mansions feel to ruin,
 And the palaces to decay.
And the lonely, silent child,
 Sat in isolated play.

Until nothing was left,
 Of the boy inside.
And no palace of dreams,
 Where one could hide.

But when manhood came.
 As manhood will.
The lonely boy,
 Tried hiding still.

In the land of lies,
 In the land of dreams.
A boy survives,
 Or so it seems.

By: Don Moore

MISSING PIECES

I stumbled upon an empty space that occupies my soul
My feelings, thoughts and emotions from each it exacts a toll
Reminding me with every sign of isolation dark face

The feeling that this piece I lack suspends me in time and space

This item that I speak of, one can neither see nor touch
Inconspicuous in its absence but without it life lacks so much
If only I could buy it, this commodity for which I seek
To stop this insidious gnawing that for years has left me weak

The depth of my own neediness I did not wish to know
Somehow I'll just get better and never face that foe
So I skirt recovery's fringes with my guard kept well in tact
But as it is with all such lies truth seeks out the smallest crack

It could not come with thunder when that ray of truth broke through
But in it crept so softly with this conclusion it lead me too
I ran along behind this truth fingers groping in the dark
Ever fearful I might catch a glimpse of that elusive missing part

When its face did finally show itself my fears at once came true
The face my own, this message brings first seek this piece in you
Darkness closed around me like a blanket pulled over my

head
I have always sought out others to revive in me what's dead

With now the truth stripped naked as I gaze inside my heart
I see within what's missing a fundamental basic part
The structure always crumbles for it lacks this cornerstone
No happiness from within me and that peace I seek on Loan

Perry Moore
Oct., 1993

DREAMS

A poet's touch is what I need,
And I'd be something, yes indeed!
For when I write these things I feel,
It comes to me as very real.

If only, I was someone other than me,
Then I might surely have the vision to see,
That these things I need are simple and nice,
A home, a wife and a real happy life.

And as I write this I feel a tear,
For what I need I really fear!
These needs, these fears, such thoughts of mine,
Could make me the poet of my dreams in time.

And this at first, I could not believe,
That it's me the poet of the dreams I conceived.

N. Lieberman
1957

DIVIDED WHY?

Why O' why must men be born,
Such one is white and one is dark?
And in between the two shall know,
An insurmountable barrier of class.

Why O' G-d has thou conceived,
the domination of one of thine?
And in this world of divided minds,
How will mankind survive this plan?

For until the two can live side by side,
Peace on earth is doomed forever!
And who must bear the responsibility,
For such a catastrophe happening here?

And then I asked the One who knows,
And only silence did I hear!

N. Lieberman
1957

YOU CAN SUCCEED AT ANYTHING

NEVER LOOK BACK
FIND A ROLE MODEL

View problems as challenges you can overcome
Review your past successes to help you

When distracting thoughts come to mind say to yourself STOP, then close your eyes take a deep breath. Hold until the count of three. As you exhale think to yourself, relax and let go. Focus all your energy on one thought ---the job ahead of you.

Watch the calendar instead of the clock. The self disciplined person doesn't measure time with a stopwatch but with a calendar, planning a series of small triumphs that may take weeks or months as a way of reaching an ultimate goal.

Use positive thinking. Put failure out of your mind and replace with thoughts of success, how to succeed what to do next, you'll move in the direction of your thoughts.

Use creative day dreaming. What is it you want your self discipline to help you accomplish? Draw a picture in your mind of exactly what things will be like when you achieve your goal.

Plan ways to succeed in small goals.
Don't try to be perfect. Praise yourself for thinking each step.

Keep balance in your life, you know when to play as well as when to work. Life is divided into three major components: work, play and love. Don't ignore anyone of them or you'll be sitting on a three-legged stool.

Bill Ullian

ONE LONG NIGHT

It was late and I was pacing
And my mind was ill at ease
Just to keep my thoughts from racing
I went walking through the trees
And in the middle of a clearing
I looked for a soul to save
In a ring of stones appearing
To contain a shallow grave
But there the ground was cold and ashen
Where a living flame once burned
Full of promise and of passion
And unto dust returned.

One long night,
It has been one long night..

I have come though I grow weary
Looking for the light,
Trying with all my might.
It has been one long night,
One long night.

So I sat for countless hours
Stirring cinders in the dark,
Hoping for my sleeping powers
To awaken with a spark.
Once I set the world on fire
then I was consumed by doubt,
Soon I felt my heart's desire
Gradually burning out.
But if I find a glowing ember
Buried in these grey remains,
I am old but I remember
How to start again.

One long night,
It has been one long night.
I won't rest until I see me
Standing in the light.
Then it'll be alright.
It has been one long night.
One long night.

Joe Allen

OUR GARDEN

Do not sleep while there's still light
On the threshold of the night.
Soon, I pray, will come the hour
When our garden starts to flower.
All is not despair and doom.
There is time enough to bloom.
Never let us give up hoping.
Keep your weary eyes wide open.

Love is a lesson that's never too late;
Counting our blessings and learning to wait;
Looking for beauty in all we create;
Love is a lesson that's never too late.
Love is a lesson that's never too late.
And all the seeds that we have planted
Deeply in the earth,
Labor there a little longer
'Til the moment of their birth.

Good things come to those who see.
Endless possibility.
Love will come at any minute
Won't be long before we're in it.
You will see beyond a doubt
We'll be glad we stuck it out.
Every petal is preparing

For the joy that we'll be sharing.

There's a great expectancy
Growing in its certainty.
Patience now and in good measure
We will reap a living treasure.
Though the ground is hard and grey,
Keep believing in today.
Faith is power, pure and awesome,
Every bud is bound to blossom.

Joe Allen
1996

INNER CHILD

Little girl, inside my heart,
I turned away right from the start,
Frightened of your pain so deep,
And all the secrets you do keep.

I see you crying all alone,
No place is safe, not even home,
You look at me, eyes full of fear,
I pull you close and keep you near.

I say, "I love you, you're safe now",
As I softly stroke your brow,

And rock you gently till you sleep,
You feel my love, so warm and deep.

Still some days I run away,
But please have patience for some day,
I'll reach for you and hold you tight,
Protect and love you, day and night.

I'll keep you always in my heart,
And never will we be apart,
We'll feel our pain, will understand,
And walk life's road, hand in hand.

I'll look at me with eyes that see,
The love I have inside of me,
For the young girl in my heart,
Has been me right from the start.

Debra C. Jermyn and all parts of the whole

May, 1991

FRAGMENTS

Blonde-haired girl, alone and small,
"He" comes slowly down the hall.
Crying quietly on the floor,
She can't take it anymore.

Terror fills her sad green eyes,
Then he laughs and tells her lies,
"I won't hurt you" he softly said,
As he placed her on the bed.

Her body feels, her mind is cold,
At the age of six, she is very old.
His eyes are blank, his body steel,
Another part of her comes to feel.

She plays above the bed today,
With others who have gone away.
Love and comfort they do give,
So the blonde-haired girl can live.

The lies were told, the damage done,
To the little girl so young.
The tears are gone, the feelings lost,
She paid the price at any cost.

Wanting to be whole once more,
No key found for the locked, closed door.
Time and love and hope may find,
The key that's lost inside her mind.

Debra C. Jermyn and all parts of the whole
February, 1991

CORNERS OF MY MIND

Small face and hands pressed to the door,
The reality strikes her to the core
Heart full of pain, eyes straining tears,
No love, no mommy, her greatest fears.

She waits ... in a corner of my mind.

Six years old with pain filled yes,
"No more tears" she tries but cries.
She longs for love but her soul can't feel,
Because in her world unreal is real.

She cries ... in a corner of my mind.

Child-woman, naive and sweet,
She dances away on pointed feet,
From the cold, harsh world of chance,
And dreams of princes, love and dance.

She dances ... in a corner of my mind.

Young woman laughs like all is well,
But rage and pain are her private hell.
She screams and yells and cuts and carves,
But in her heart and mind, she starves.

She is angry ... in a corner of my mind.
Mother, wife, adult and friend,
She thinks about the past to mend
With intellect, reason and logical thought,
Can't comprehend why the feelings stay caught.
She thinks ... in a corner of my mind.
In the corners of my mind,
Are all the parts I need to find,
For all of "me" to grow and heal,
Forgive and love and live and feel.
We are together ... in my mind.

Debra C. Jermyn and all parts of the whole
Oct. 1991

SHADES OF GREY

In between the good and bad,
In between the glad and sad,
Are the shades and hues of grey,
We learn to live with everyday.

Grey has many names, you know,
Light black, silver, trodden snow,
White and black mixed through and through,
so many shades make me and you.

You say you wear a hat of grey,

Not black, not white, no how, no way!
See your good, your bad, see you,
You are many, not just two.

So here's a small reminder of,
The color grey I've grown to love,
And the wonder grey can be,
When you care enough to see.

Debra C. Jermyn and all parts of the whole
Dec., 1991

IN MEMORY OF JOE BROWN FEBRUARY 6, 1997

THERE'S ONE LESS BEAR IN THE ROOM TONIGHT

There's one less bear
in the room tonight
just an old brown teddy
you could hold so tight.

A gentle bear
with dark brown eyes
who helped our laughter
and comforted our cries.

Just a raggedy old bear
with a heart so true
he knew your troubles
and he knew mine too.

But he's been called
away to a place
a place of beauty
and a place of grace.

So, with his friend
dear Joe Brown
they're two fine bears
out on the town.

But there's one less bear
on the room tonight
and a new star shinning
in the heavens bright.

Don Moore
February 12, 1997

"When one door of happiness closes, another opens; but often we look so long at the closed door that we do not see the one that has been opened for us."

Helen Keller

Chapter IX

Special Comminications

To G-d
To Little Rachel
To my therapist
From my therapist
To my surgeon
To my family of choice
To you, the reader

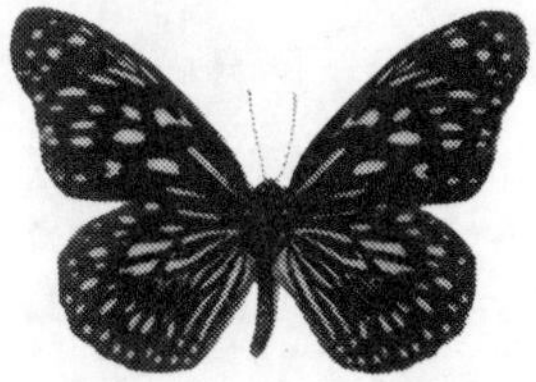

B"H
July 6, 1993

Dear G-d,

I never realized that you had given me so many gifts in this life. One by one in recovery they began to surface and I could no longer deny that they were there from the very start 53 years ago! Your first gift to me was life itself and although it did not feel like a gift for the first five decades it truly does three years later.

I never dreamed that I would come to realize that I am very beautiful on the inside. I never dreamed that any other human being would recognize it either. And I never dreamed that I would be able to sense it in others.

I never dreamed that I could learn to love myself and feel so wonderful on this journey. I never dreamed that I could learn to say no and to discover healthy boundaries where they were needed — give space to others when need be and to not feel disappointment at every turn. I never dreamed that I could spend a summer with myself and Little Rachel and feel so well.

And most of all I would never have imagined that I was deserving of a miracle in my life from you Dear G-d! And if all this was enough I have come to believe that I am that miracle, willing and more able to enjoy the magnificent gift of life that you gave me! I know today that I will definitely not die before I have a chance to live. Just knowing that helps me to feel anything but depressed. I can't imagine receiving greater gifts in life than these. I can imagine now feeling and being healthier and healing on your very special journey for me! For all these blessings, G-d, I am truly thankful!

Rachel

January 10, 1993

Dear Little Rachel,

It is wonderful that since I found you and know where you got stuck that we have embraced each other on this journey. We can share both our pain and happiness always! We have both grown in maturity and understanding on so many issues but this major issue of boundaries, especially with therapy, has been most challenging.

I know that issues can only be this uncomfortable and painful when we give them permission to be, in all honesty, I admit that I have perhaps done that and caused us both much discomfort. For sure, I believe that I, as the grown adult person, reflect your neediness and feelings of abandonment from our parents and projecting inappropriate behavior at times as a result.

Little Rachel, we can be stronger and take better care of ourselves. We have the most beautiful recovery friends in the world that love us dearly and will be there for us when needed. We know we have the safest place possible with our Higher Power. We have a shield of protection that can work for us always! As we begin to help others cope better with life's many stresses, we can work on our faith, our understanding and our continued growth!

Big Rachel

To My Therapist

Moore Beauty In This World

It doesn't happen overnight,
things rarely ever can,
becoming a soul healer,
is a gift from G-d, not man.

One must travel through the darkness,
and walk in that Indian's shoes,
come through the storm and find the light,
a brand new path to choose.

When all this is behind us,
on this journey we discover,
that we can find peace and balance within,
and slowly we recover.

My inner child got very stuck,
way back in my distant past,
she was very young and very scared,
and reparenting her is a challenging task.

My teacher, guide and mentor,
raised with scarcity, abuse and shame,
has helped me to understand so well,
never to judge or blame

He teaches me to appreciate life,
this only one we are given,
not to dwell in depressive thinking,
but, to let go and enjoy living.

This therapeutic, gentle man,
of whom I speak is Don Moore,
he has brought me through my darkest times,
to my Higher Power's door.

And it doesn't happen overnight,
things rarely ever can,
becoming a soul healer,
is a gift from G-d, not man.

My soul wound is closing and healing,
I feel it more every day,
and so Don, I especially salute you,
for always showing me the way!

August, 1995

DON MOORE, L.C.S.W.
Psychotherapist

Dear Rachel:

It was with great pleasure that I accepted your invitation to include a personal letter from myself to you as part of your book.

We began our journey nearly six years ago when you first came to my Wednesday night support group meeting. You sat withdrawn in the softly lit office clinging to each word and each story that was told and spoken that evening. It seemed that each person in the room was a life raft and you, the survivor holding on so that the waters of depression would not pull you under.

It was from that evening, that our individual work began with your first appointment for therapy. I marveled at your tenacity each time you came to your appointment. I could see even through your silence, the torment that shame and dysfunction from your family of origin had wreaked upon your life. Sometimes a single word or sentence was all you were able to utter in those first days. Head down, eyes averted, we struggled to develop the necessary rapport to begin your recovery.

Finally, however, the shroud of secrecy and the malaise of misery began to give way. Session by session, the story poured out, the trust developed and the growth began. Many times in our work, we have referred to the metamorphose of the butterfly. It has become the symbol for your own growth and development. Today, with the publication of your first book, you cast aside the veil of shame, and move into your rightful place as a person with her own power and sense of direction.

At last, the butterfly spreads it's wings and takes flight, its previous life not even a memory. Now as you look back over what once was, you can experience the true joy of what is today. May you enjoy success and happiness as you embrace the next phase of your growth.

Don Moore, L.C.S.W.

To My Breast Surgeon

B"H
October 21, 1993

Dear Dr. Derhagopian,

Physicians and surgeons see thousands of people in their practices throughout the years with so many various problems and issues to work through. I am just one patient in that myriad of people, but one with a special challenge to confront and overcome. I have no doubts that I can do this!

Aside from my life-long fear of medical procedures, the word cancer represented a death sentence for me whenever I heard it or saw the written word. Today, I know that this does not have to be true at all--that we can find remission with this disease and live a longer and healthier life than ever before! I have learned in my quest for emotional wellness in the past three years, that physical health without emotional wholeness will destroy the best of physical conditions in time--that our emotional health is tantamount to our over-all well being.

As I mentioned to you on the phone, I am so very grateful that G-d and Judy Sorge led me to your door. This is just one of many positive events that have been placed in my path to emotional and physical wellness in my life.

Thank you for your time and patience with me and your understanding of the space that I am coming from. I am optimistic that putting my life in your hands is the wisest thing I can do for myself come Monday morning. I am more confident than ever before that I know that you are really there to help me through this surgery experience. G-d bless you!

Respectfully,

Rachel Lieberman

B"H
December, 1994

Dear Family of Choice,

The depth and magnitude of this disease called codependency continues to boggle my mind at times, even after four years of active recovery. It took such a long time for my psyche to absorb and accept the true definition of the word. It is a transition to accept the death of the old us in exchange for a beautiful new person that emerges, when we work diligently to rise from the quagmire, to find our healthy way in recovery.

Rather, early on, the child is contaminated with the disease in the dysfunctional setting and carries those consequences throughout his life experience. Codependents never have that original chance to swim in anything but rough waters from the beginning. The challenge to stay afloat amidst the shame and confusion is given up by many who never make it to recovery's door.

And so, getting past the grief of all this is a challenge too...the grief of a lost childhood or the grief of two emotionally absent parents. And, for me, accepting that the disease is cross generational and clearly witnessing it in my three children was shocking at first also.

But, the awareness for me and my immediate family was the rainbow and the blessing after the mighty storm. The movement and energies set in motion from a power greater than myself is so awesome for this codependent. Nothing that happens for me today is terribly shocking or surprising, as in the past. I know today that G-d has a plan for me and that I am finding my way in his world to grow and change and make healthier decisions than I have ever made before.

So, when the word cancer came into my life last year, yes, the experience was devastating but my tears and fears that I had came from desperately wanting to really live now before experiencing a final transition from this world. The gift of life...of truly feeling like that free spirit that the monarch represents to me, is what I glean from the opportunity to recover from codependency. It is toward that goal that I am propelled forward and onward.

Rachel Lieberman

B"H
February, 1997

To you, the reader,

I know so well today that we do not become sick overnight and we surely don't heal overnight either! For me, the journey began when I made the commitment to exchange my very unhealthy lifestyle for one where I can find balance, focus and some inner peace.

I have found a good measure of that serenity with my connectedness to a spiritual universal force that I choose to call G-d! I have found my faith on this path that has helped me to let go of monumental and catastrophic fear that had crippled me all my life!

I could do none of this alone. Exceptional therapy, support groups and other professionals helped me and my child to climb each mountain. G-d opened each new door as I was ready to accept each challenge. I am so proud to be a recovering person today!

I am finding happiness with myself and others. I am feeling more empowered to live life to its fullest! Today, after six years, I know and understand the reality of my codependent disease. The more I do know and understand, the better I can accept the responsibility of working to remain as strong and as healthy as I can be in the moment, in the hour and for the day! I wish all of you, my readers, the same blessing on your journeys!

Yours in recovery,

Rachel Lieberman

"This above all: To thine own self be true, and it must follow, as the night the day, thou cannot be false to any man."

Shakespeare

Chapter X

A Closing Word

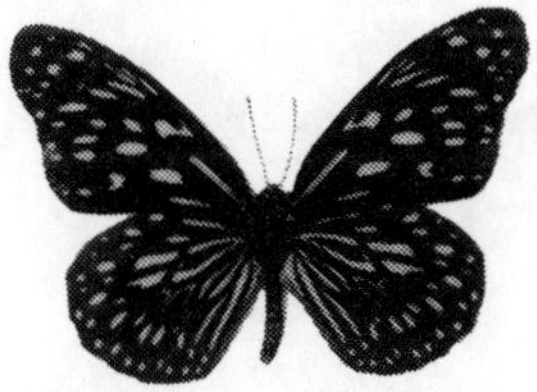

Chapter X

A Closing Word

Codependents are special people. We are G-d's healing army. We are the walking wounded, working to heal our souls! Our needs are great because we were deprived perhaps not only of the material necessities of life but of the nurturing and loving and boding that we so hungered for in our pasts. We still desperately need them all in the present. We no longer have to sit at the banquet table and starve! We can make a lifetime commitment to be emotionally well!

In recovery, we can mirror healthier behaviors that we are proud of to our families and friends. It is not too late to be our true and beautiful selves. It is not too late for our inner child to emerge and be free. We can feel whole and serene on the journey. We can make a difference to ourselves, our families and friends, our support team and program and also to our family of choice.

My personal world has changed considerably in the past six years! I am no longer lost. I am feeling the glow of more wellness. I feel the miracle and the metamorphosis as I continue to work on my self spiritually, emotionally and physically!

I would venture to say that this disease of codependency is

probably one of the most negative forces in the universe! It saturates and seeps into every corner of the earth and is at the core of many of the atrocities that demonstrates man's inhumanity to man! It is rampant and unharnessed for the most part and is so harmfully dangerous! It is reality! For all of us who are fortunate enough to get a handle on this enemy and find refuge and peace in our lives, recovery is salvation. I would be surprised if it were possible to statistically know how many people in this world have not been touched in some way with codependency. I am sure that it would be quite a low percentage indeed!

The recovery experts talk about that "family trance" that people live in. Certainly our parents, our grandparents and the generations before them were most likely born, raised and died, never emerging from this fog. There were very few opportunities for them to get psychological guidance in their lives and they experienced the emptiness, the ongoing feelings of low self-esteem hiding in addictions and exhibiting strong behaviors of control, anger and rage! They never discovered where these were coming from or why this was all happening for them. My European father was a pure example!

I believe that perhaps the new age of enlightenment might have begun with the invention of the television set and the mass communication of satellite broadcasting! The world began pouring into our living rooms, especially in recent years with the introduction of the "talk show"! They broke the ice for candid discussion about any issue under the sun! These daily opportunities today can trigger awareness for so many in that trance state today!

My gratitude for this beautiful journey of healing did not begin with a talk show but with another hurting human being extending love and caring to me. I realized early on that I did not have to remain in this sick state all my life and be a party to constant pain and suffering with addictions and very low self-esteem. I discovered that I could feel more real like that famous velveteen rabbit and enjoy a real life. It has been a long six year journey from then until now! Today, I am not just surviving, I am thriving! I can both laugh and cry now at appropriate times. I can work on my issues with openness and honesty, experiencing and accepting all of life's stages and not allowing them to devastate me. I am beautiful inside and out. I am sure of it. I am me and only me. I am very okay and I say yes to life!

Order Form

Telephone orders: Call: 1-(561) 338-9108

Postal orders: My Inner Child Creations
Rachel Lieberman, Suite 144, 3840 W.
Hillsboro Blvd., Deerfield Beach, Fl 33442
Tel: 1-561-338-9108
@ $13.95

Please send me ____ copies of A Leaf Falls..
A Bud Blossoms

Name: ______________________________

Address: ____________________________

City: __________ State: ______ Zip: _______

Telephone: (___) ____________________

Payment:
Send money order or check payable to:
My Inner Child Creations

Allow 3 to 5 weeks for delivery.

Sales Tax:
Please add 6% for books shipped in Florida.

Shipping and Handling:
$3.00 for the first book and $1.00 for each additional book

ORDER NOW

Name

Address

Sales

Shipping and handling

ORDER NOW

Order Form

Telephone orders: Call: 1-(561) 338-9108

Postal orders: My Inner Child Creations
Rachel Lieberman, Suite 144, 3840 W.
Hillsboro Blvd., Deerfield Beach, Fl 33442
Tel: 1-561-338-9108
@ $13.95

Please send me ____ copies of A Leaf Falls..
A Bud Blossoms

Name: ______________________________

Address: ____________________________

City: __________ State: ______ Zip: _______

Telephone: (___) ______________________

Payment:
Send money order or check payable to:
My Inner Child Creations

Allow 3 to 5 weeks for delivery.

Sales Tax:
Please add 6% for books shipped in Florida.

Shipping and Handling:
$3.00 for the first book and $1.00 for each additional book

ORDER NOW

Order Form